Checklist
for Your
First Baby

Checklist

for Your

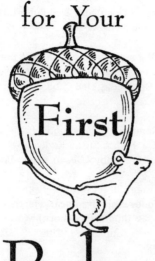

First

Baby

Susan Kagen Podell, M.S., R.D.

Main Street Books
Doubleday
New York London Toronto Sydney Auckland

A MAIN STREET BOOK

PUBLISHED BY DOUBLEDAY

a division of Bantam Doubleday Dell Publishing Group, Inc.
1540 Broadway, New York, New York 10036

MAIN STREET BOOKS, DOUBLEDAY, and the portrayal of a
building with a tree are trademarks of Doubleday, a division
of Bantam Doubleday Dell Publishing Group, Inc.

Library of Congress Cataloging-in-Publication Data
Podell, Susan Kagen.
Checklist for your first baby / Susan Kagen Podell. — 1st ed.
p.   cm.
"A Main Street Book"—T.p. verso.
Includes bibliographical references.
1. Pregnancy.   2. Infants (Newborn)—Care.   3. Infants'
supplies.   I. Title.
RG525.P58   1997
618.2′4—dc20   96-11909
                                                              CIP

ISBN 0-385-47797-X

BOOK DESIGN BY CAROL MALCOLM RUSSO/
SIGNET M DESIGN, INC.

Printed in the United States of America
February 1997
3   5   7   9   10   8   6   4
FIRST EDITION

To my wonderful husband, Michael,
whose love and support
helped make this book a reality;
and to my two beautiful daughters,
Rachel and Dana,
whose very existence provided
my inspiration.

Contents

Contents

Introduction

Congratulations! You're expecting a baby—one of life's most joyful experiences. The next nine months will be a flurry of changes and a whirlwind of activity that will bring challenges, excitement, and many questions.

Checklist for Your First Baby has been designed to help you through all phases of these changes—physical, emotional, and especially logistical. New parenthood can make you apprehensive, but it's really fear of the unknown. With this book as your all-in-one planning resource, you will be organized and ready when the big day arrives! You can use the pregnancy calendar for quick, easy reference, and the memorable keepsakes section for memories of your baby's first hours and days of life. Your body is expanding as your time seems to be shrinking. Use the information, lists, and reminders in this book to check off the challenges of pregnancy and new parenthood one step, one task, at a time.

How to Use This Book

Checklist for Your First Baby is divided into four parts, one for each of the three trimesters and one for the weeks following birth. A pregnancy calendar is also included. Read each part at the appropriate time and use the information and checklists to make sure you're on schedule. You don't need to read ahead since all tasks are ordered during the correct trimester. Sometimes completing a task too early means you'll have to redo it later. Keep the book in a handy place and bring it with you to all prenatal health visits and maternity or baby shopping excursions. If you are already pregnant, you can start using the book immediately. If you're planning a pregnancy, use the health and nutrition information to give your baby the best head start possible.

How to Use This Book

Checklist
for Your
First Baby

Section One:
How You and Your Baby Grow and Change

As you move through your pregnancy, you'll notice many changes going on in and outside your body. Some of these changes will be physical and therefore visible to the world. But some will be emotional—feelings only you and, if you share them, your partner, will know. It's a beautiful time, full of hopes, wishes, and dreams. In the first few months, however, you may feel frustrated or confused. Although you know you're pregnant, you can't actually see the changes that are happening and all you want to do is sleep. Take heart! As the weeks and months progress, your energy levels will return. Your waistline will slowly disappear and soon you'll begin to wear maternity clothes. You'll experience the thrilling feeling of life inside you for the first time and begin to notice changes in your breasts, which are preparing to feed a new life. Be patient. The profound and wonderful changes that are pregnancy will happen to you in due course. Relax and enjoy one of the most amazing years of your life!

The following is a guide to help you antipate what you may be feeling and ho baby is developing during the nine months, or forty weeks, of pregnancy.

THE FIRST TRIMESTER
(Weeks One to Twelve)

Month 1

At the end of your fourth week of pregnancy, your baby is about ½ inch long and weighs less than one ounce. On day twenty-five your baby's heart is beating and the brain, backbone, spinal cord, and digestive system are also forming. Small buds that will eventually become arms and legs are present.

Your body is going through many changes also. You've missed a period or may have spotty bleeding instead of a normal period. You may feel nauseated with or without vomiting due to an increase in hormone production. These symptoms, known as morning sickness, can actually occur any time of the day or night. Nausea also may recur in later months, when your baby is pressing on your stomach. To help prevent and treat morning sickness, try the following: Eat small, frequent light meals and snacks. Nausea becomes worse when the stomach is empty. Eat plenty of starchy foods such as bread, pasta, rice, and potatoes. Avoid greasy icy foods and foods with strong smells. Eat cold foods and drink cold liquids, as these seem to be better tolerated than hot items. Keep crackers, popcorn, dry cereal, or graham crackers by your bed. Eating something when you first wake up may help prevent or relieve nausea. Avoid sudden movements upon arising, and choose foods high in Vitamin B_6—such as kidney beans, chicken, brussels sprouts, bananas, potatoes, lean hamburger, and sunflower seeds—which according to a recent study by the University of Iowa College of Medicine can relieve nausea in pregnant women.

You will notice at this time that your breasts are also changing. They are larger than usual, tender, and your nipples are more prominent.

Month 2

By the end of your eighth week of pregnancy the baby is about 1⅛ inches long and still weighs less than one ounce. The face and features are forming, but the eyelids are fused shut. Limbs are beginning to show distinct divisions into upper arms, elbows, forearms, and hands, and thighs, knees, lower legs, and feet. Internal organs and long bones are developing. A distinct umbilical cord is formed and the placenta is now nourishing your baby.

Your breasts may still feel tender or lumpy, and often tingling or throbbing occurs. Your uterus is now soft and about the size of a tennis ball. To protect your baby, a mucous plug forms at the mouth of your cervix. You will probably feel tired and need extra sleep.

Month 3

At the end of twelve weeks your baby is about three to four inches long and weighs about one ounce. Its arms, hands, fingers, legs, feet, and toes are fully formed. Fingernails and toenails are developing and ears are present. Twenty tooth buds are forming in the jaw. The eyes are almost fully developed, but still fused shut. External sex organs begin to indicate if your baby is a boy or a girl. Your baby can now kick, make a fist, turn its head, frown, and squint.

Morning sickness usually disappears at the end of this month and your energy level may return. Your uterus is now the size of an orange and your waistline is disappearing as your baby grows. Now is a good time to begin sharing your wonderful news with others.

THE SECOND TRIMESTER
(Weeks Thirteen to Twenty-four)

Month 4

By the end of the sixteenth week, your baby is about 6½ to 7 inches long and weighs four to five ounces. It has a strong heartbeat, moves, kicks, sleeps and wakes, swallows, and can pass urine. Its skin is bright pink, transparent, and covered with a fine downlike hair called lanugo. Your baby has eyebrows and a small amount of hair on its head as well as vocal cords and taste buds.

You are now starting to look pregnant with your uterus the size of a grapefruit. A yellowish-white fluid called colostrum may leak from your nipples. This is normal. It's your body's way of preparing for nursing once your baby is born. Colostrum is the first fluid a breastfeeding baby eats. It's rich in nutrients and antibodies to help fight infections. The area around your nipple, the areola, becomes darker and larger, and small bumps appear in preparation for milk production. You may now begin to feel the baby move. Quickening, as it is called, may feel like small bubbles or the fluttering of wings. A smaller woman may notice quickening earlier than a larger woman. Tell your health care provider when you first feel fetal movement, as this can help confirm your due date.

Month 5
At the end of twenty weeks, your baby measures approximately eight to twelve inches and weighs 1/2 to one pound. The internal organs are maturing rapidly, but the lungs are not fully developed. Your baby is now doing lots of kicking, turning from side to side, and rolling head over heels. Your baby sleeps and wakes at regular

intervals, has hair, can suck its thumb and get hiccups.

Your uterus has expanded to reach the height of your navel and the skin on your abdomen stretches. You may become constipated because of pressure on the lower intestine from the enlarging uterus. Usually between the eighteenth and twentieth week your health care provider will be able to hear your baby's heartbeat—you'll be able to hear that miraculous sound too!

Month 6
By the end of twenty-four weeks your baby measures eleven to fourteen inches and weighs one to 1½ pounds. Its skin is quite wrinkled, reddish in color, and covered with a heavy protective coating called vernix. Your baby can now open and close its eyes and hear sounds inside you. Eyelashes and unique fingerprints and footprints have formed.

You may feel the baby kicking high in your abdomen or low near your bladder. Frequent urges to urinate are common. You may also experience a stitch like pain down the side of your abdomen as the uterine muscles stretch. Stretch marks may develop on your abdomen, breasts, or thighs. Don't be alarmed, after delivery these marks will slowly fade.

THE THIRD TRIMESTER
(Weeks Twenty-five to Forty)

Month 7

After twenty-eight weeks the baby's weight has about doubled since the last month to 2½ to three pounds and it's about three inches longer, at about fifteen inches. It still looks reddish and wrinkled. The wrinkles will eventually be filled with "baby fat" by the middle of the eighth month. Your baby exercises by kicking and stretching. The centers of the baby's bones are hardening.

You may develop hemorrhoids, swollen blood vessels in the rectum, and may experience discomfort during bowel movements. False labor pains called Braxton Hicks contractions, may be felt every so often. They usually feel like strong menstrual cramps. Also at this time you may experience a range of new emotions. Mood swings including feelings of elation and doubt are not unusual. Fear or apprehension about labor, delivery, and motherhood are common, and it's normal for you to want your pregnancy to be over.

Month 8

The baby matures a lot in the last two months of pregnancy. It will add two to 2½ more pounds and grow to sixteen to eighteen inches long. Movements or kicks may actually be seen from the outside of your body and are felt much more strongly. Although your baby's bones continue to harden, the bones of the head are soft and flexible. Your baby can now hear sounds outside your body.

You may find yourself short of breath and feeling aches and pains in your back, abdomen, and groin. Your contractions may be stronger and colostrum may begin to leak, if it hasn't been leaking already from your breasts. Sleeping may be difficult since it's hard to find a comfortable position. Lying on your left side with one leg crossed over you may help you sleep better, or try placing a pillow between your legs in this position for extra comfort.

Month 9

At full term your baby weighs about seven to 7½ pounds and measures about twenty inches long. Your baby is fully developed with smooth skin. The baby has a "soft spot" on its head to allow for delivery. When ready to be born, your baby will drop down into your pelvis and engage itself in the birth position.

You will find breathing easier once the baby has dropped, but since it is now pressing against your bladder you may once again have to urinate frequently. Often leaning forward while urinating will make passing urine easier. During this time your cervix will soften and contractions will increase. Often the colostrum leaking from your nipples increases and you may want to use breast pads to avoid soiling your bras. You may feel tired, anxious, tense, and elated. Weekly visits to your health care provider will help ease your anxiety, as will the continued love and support of your partner, family, and friends. Your baby is now ready to be born!

Section Two:
What to Do the
First Trimester

THREE STEPS TO A HEALTHY BABY

Your health during your pregnancy directly affects the health of your baby. The healthier you are, the better are your chances of having a problem-free pregnancy, labor, and delivery. Now is the time to take charge of your health and do everything you can to give your baby a great start in life. Three important steps toward this goal are proper medical care, good nutrition, and appropriate exercise.

Step One: Proper Medical Care

Regular medical care by a physician or certified nurse-midwife should begin as soon as you suspect you are pregnant. Your health care provider is the best person to confirm your pregnancy and get you and your baby off to a healthy start. There are three types of practitioners you can choose to take care of you while you are pregnant. They all differ in their medical credentials and philosophy of practice.

The Ob-Gyn, or Obstetrician   Obstetricians are specialists trained to handle all possible emergencies and complications associated with childbirth. The overwhelming majority of women choose this type of doctor to care for them during pregnancy, labor, and delivery. If your pregnancy is high risk, or if you are under seventeen or over thirty-five, you'll probably want to choose this type of practitioner. Even if your pregnancy is pretty routine, you wouldn't be alone if you chose an ob-gyn to care for you.

The Family Practice Physician   The family practitioner is a medical specialty similar in many ways to the old-fashioned general practitioner. This physician is specially trained in primary care, including obstetrics. A family practice doctor can be your physician before, during, and after your pregnancy and can be the pediatrician for your baby as well. The family practitioner is usually familiar with all aspects of your health and your family situation. He or she will treat your pregnancy as a normal part of life rather than an illness, but will often consult with an ob-gyn if complications do occur.

The Certified Nurse-Midwife   In addition to being registered nurses, certified nurse-midwives have spent one to two more years of training in clinical midwifery skills. They not only can supervise childbirth, they also are trained in prenatal and well-women care, including gynecological exams, pap smears, and contraceptive, lactation, and menopause education. Midwives view pregnancy as a normal, healthy process. They tend to take a low-tech approach to childbirth and to treat their patients as people first rather than sick individuals in need of care. If you choose a midwife, be sure she's certified. Remember that midwives are trained to handle only low-risk, uncomplicated pregnancies.

During your nine months of pregnancy your health care provider will schedule a series of appointments—once a month for the first few months and more often later on, often weekly during the last four to eight weeks. It's a good idea to keep a written schedule of your medical appointments. Use the pregnancy calendar at the end of this book for that purpose.

Remember, you are a partner with your health care provider. The information you provide will help him or her take better care of you. No question is too silly or unimportant to ask, and no unusual symptom should go unreported. It's helpful to keep a running list of nonemergency questions between each appointment. Use the following checklist of questions as a starting point. Bring this book, your list of questions, and a pen with you to all prenatal visits.

✓ ✓ ✓ ✓ ✓ ✓ ✓ ✓ ✓ ✓ ✓ ✓ ✓ ✓ ✓

Checklist of Questions for Your Health Care Provider

○ **1.** Are there any restrictions on travel? working? lovemaking?

○ **2.** Are there any restrictions on food?

○ **3.** What are your feelings on caffeinated and alcoholic beverages in moderation? What, if any, is an acceptable amount?

○ **4.** Are there any restrictions on prescription or over-the-counter medications?

○ **5.** Do I need a prenatal vitamin? If so, when should I start taking it?

○ **6.** Should I take precautions concerning pets or household cleaning supplies?

○ **7.** Which hospitals are you affiliated with and which ones do you suggest I tour?

○ **8.** Where and when can I enroll in childbirth preparation classes? Are there any other educational classes I should take?

○ **9.** Will I need any special tests?

○ **10.** What happens if you are not available when I go into labor?

○ **11.** When should I call you when I am in labor?

○ **12.** Where do I go in an emergency?

○ **13.** What is your attitude about pain relief during labor? What about natural childbirth?

○ **14.** What is your attitude about fetal monitoring? induced labor? episiotomies? C-sections? squatting during delivery? walking during labor?

○ **15.** What role do you feel the father should play during childbirth, including C-sections?

If you have a problem that requires immediate attention, make sure you call your health care provider as soon as possible. Use the following tips as a guide when calling:

1. Make the call yourself if at all possible. No one can describe your symptoms as well as you can.

2. Be specific when describing your problem. Include a description of the symptoms, when they began, how long they have continued, and the part of your body that is affected.

3. If the problem occurs when your health care provider cannot be reached (for example, when the office is closed), go directly to the hospital and ask the hospital staff to contact your health care provider.

Notify your health care provider immediately if you experience any of the following symptoms during pregnancy:

1. A sudden increase or change in vaginal discharge

2. Any vaginal bleeding

3. Five or more contractions in an hour (contractions may not be painful, they could just involve tightening and relaxing of the uterus, which can be felt by placing your hand on your abdomen)

4. Menstrual-like cramps or pelvic pressure

5. Persistent diarrhea or intestinal cramps

6. A low, dull backache that doesn't improve with rest

7. A general feeling that something is wrong

Remember to get plenty of rest and minimal stress. Try sleeping seven to eight hours a night and nap when possible on weekends. Also try to avoid anything that causes a large amount of stress. It's stressful enough making the adjustment to being pregnant without additional worries!

Vital Statistics Checklist

Prepregnancy weight:
First day of last menstrual period:
Expected due date:
Mom's blood type:
    Rh factor:
Dad's blood type:
    Rh factor:

Step Two: Good Nutrition: What You Eat Is What You Get

Pregnancy can be one of the most exciting times of your life. It is also a time of change. You begin taking care of your baby the moment he or she is conceived. The rapid growth and development of your baby from conception to birth demands that you provide the right foods in the right amount throughout your pregnancy, when vitamins, minerals, proteins, carbohydrates, and fats are transferred to the baby through your blood. Your nutritional health will play a major role in your ability to nourish and deliver a healthy baby.

Weight Gain: How Much Is Enough?

Ideally, you should gain twenty-four to thirty-five pounds during the nine months of pregnancy. Your health care provider will use your height, weight before you became pregnant, and frame size to determine the exact amount. If you were over- or underweight prior to pregnancy, your health care provider may recommend that you gain less or more weight than the average. You should *never* try to lose weight while you are pregnant.

In the first three months you may gain only two to four pounds, but during the next six months you can expect to gain just about one pound per week. The following chart shows how the average weight gain during pregnancy is distributed:

Baby	7.7 pounds
Placenta	1.4 pounds
Amniotic and other fluids	4.5 pounds
Increased blood volume	4.0 pounds
Uterus	2.0 pounds
Breasts	0.9 pounds
Fat stores	3.5 pounds
TOTAL	**24 pounds**

Although most women wish that fat stores did not accumulate during pregnancy, they actually serve a vital function. The few extra pounds from fat that develop during pregnancy are used after pregnancy to help women produce rich, nourishing breast milk. Even if you don't breast-feed, these few pounds can be easily lost with a healthy eating plan and exercise after your baby is born. Usually, problems losing these pounds occur only if a woman gains much more than the average. If you follow the healthy eating guidelines in this section, you'll not only nourish your baby during your pregnancy but be back to your old size in no time after your baby is born!

Although many women worry about gain-ing weight during pregnancy, don't worry until after the baby is born about losing the weight you gain. It is dangerous for the baby if you gain too little weight or lose weight, as this can lead to low birth weight and other birth problems. Remember, you will probably lose twelve to fourteen pounds within a month after delivery. With low-fat eating and exercise, the rest of the pregnancy weight gain will disappear in three to twelve months. However, if you plan to breast-feed, you will continue to need increased calories and protein until after you wean your baby because your baby will still be dependent on your food consumption for his or her nutritional needs.

During the last three months of pregnancy many women have a slight accumulation of fluid in their body. This is normal. A sudden, large weight gain, however, is not and may be a warning signal of toxemia in pregnancy. The symptoms of toxemia include an excessive and rapid buildup of fluid, high blood pressure, and protein in the urine. If you think this is happening to you, contact your health care provider immediately.

When you're pregnant, you're like an athlete in training for the big race. During the forty weeks of pregnancy a lot of energy is burned. Calories are essential. Make sure you're getting the right kind of calories—lots of complex carbohydrates like bread, cereal, rice, pasta, and

CHART YOUR WEIGHT GAIN

Plot the number of pounds gained using the left side of the graph. Plot the number of weeks pregnant using the bottom of the graph. Draw a curve as in the example.

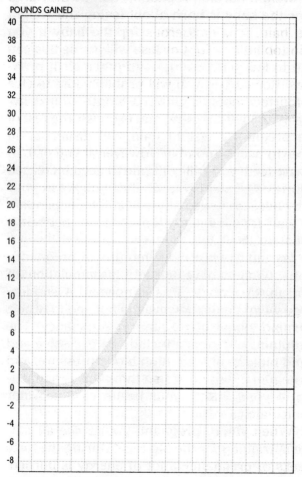

POUNDS GAINED

40
38
36
34
32
30
28
26
24
22
20
18
16
14
12
10
8
6
4
2
0
-2
-4
-6
-8

2 4 6 8 10 12 14 16 18 20 22 24 26 28 30 32 34 36 38 40
WEEKS OF PREGNANCY

potatoes to provide fuel and fiber; adequate protein from lean meats, skinless chicken, fish, and low-fat dairy foods to aid in building new cells; calcium-rich dairy products to support developing bones and teeth, and vitamin- and mineral-rich fruits and vegetables to regulate body processes. Choosing enough of the right foods every day is the best way to eat for two.

Eating Checklist for Mommies-to-Be

Complete the food checklist daily to make sure that you and your baby are getting the nutrients you both need. An extra serving of milk and meat are needed in the last trimester to provide the additional nutrition required for the last growth spurt before birth.

Another way to look at the food groups is the Food Guide Pyramid developed in 1992 by the United States Department of Agriculture. The pyramid visually focuses on the proportion of foods you need to eat rather than exact amounts. During pregnancy, even though you need more food, the proportion of food containing fats and sugars should remain small while carbohydrate foods like grains, fruits, and vegetables should be increased. The precise number of servings you should eat each day from each food group depends on how many calories you need. Ask your health care provider whether you need more or less than the average amount of 2200 calories per day.

Food Group	Servings per Day
Milk Major source of calcium and protein	3 to 4 A serving is one cup milk/yogurt or one ounce cheese.
Meat Major source of protein and iron	3 to 4 A serving is two ounces lean red meat, chicken, fish, or shellfish.
Fruits Major source of vitamins and minerals. Choose two Vitamin-C-rich sources per day.	3 or more A serving is one cup fresh, 1/2 cup cooked, 1/2 cup juice, or one medium piece.
Vegetables Major source of vitamins and minerals. Choose one Vitamin-A-rich source several times per week.	4 or more A serving is one cup fresh, 1/2 cup cooked, or 1/2 cup juice.
Breads and Cereals Major source of fiber, B vitamins, and energy	9 or more A serving is one slice of bread, one roll, 1/2 cup cooked cereal, pasta, or rice, or 1 ounce ready-to-eat cereal.

The pyramid divides food in to major groups: the bread group, the fruit group, the vegetable group, the meat group, the milk group, and fats, oils, and sweets. The base of the pyramid is the bread group. This group includes foods that come from grains, such as bread, rice, cereal, and pasta. In the same way that the bread group is the base of the pyramid, the bread group should also be the base of your diet. You need six to eleven servings of these foods per day. The next level includes foods that come from plants—the fruit and vegetable groups. They are good sources of vitamins, minerals, and fiber and are naturally low in fat. You should eat two to four servings from the fruit group and three to five servings from the vegetable group per day. The milk and meat groups comprise the next level of the pyramid. Most of the foods in these groups come from animals and are important sources of protein, iron, calcium, and zinc. Because these foods can be high in fat, it is important to make low-fat choices whenever possible. During pregnancy and lactation you need three to four servings each from the meat group and the milk group each day. The small tip of the pyramid consists of the foods that should be eaten sparingly or in small amounts. Pregnancy is *not* the time to load up on sugars and fats. You want to get the three hundred extra calories you need each day from the other categories of food in the pyramid.

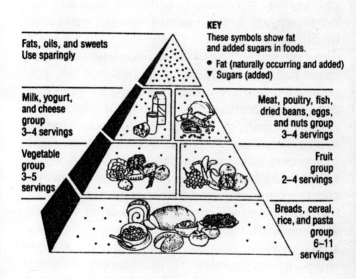

KEY

These symbols show fat and added sugars in foods.

- Fat (naturally occurring and added)
- ▼ Sugars (added)

Fats, oils, and sweets
Use sparingly

Milk, yogurt, and cheese group
3–4 servings

Meat, poultry, fish, dried beans, eggs, and nuts group
3–4 servings

Vegetable group
3–5 servings

Fruit group
2–4 servings

Breads, cereal, rice, and pasta group
6–11 servings

If you're confused about which foods pack the biggest nutritional punch, here are some guidelines that should help. Remember, you and your baby are like a team sharing all available resources. When you eat well, your baby eats well. But when you make poor food choices or skip meals, neither you nor your baby gets the nourishment you both need.

Protein: The "Building Blocks" of Life

Protein is the basic building material for you and your baby. During pregnancy your need for protein is increased. Protein is required to repair, maintain, and build new body tissue; create antibodies to fight infection; and make hormones to sustain your pregnancy. According to the Food and Nutrition Board of the National Academy of Sciences—National Research Council, the recommended dietary allowance (RDA) for protein during pregnancy is sixty grams per day. This represents a minimum. Many health care providers and registered dietitians feel that protein intake should be higher, from seventy-five to ninety grams per day.

Protein is found in a variety of foods, especially animal sources such as beef, lamb, pork, veal, poultry, fish, eggs, and dairy products. These animal sources are called complete proteins because they can build body tissue. Some vegetable or plant foods also contain protein, but this protein is incomplete since it cannot form body tissue. Incomplete protein foods need to be combined with other plant or animal foods to form tissue-building protein. The following table provides information on both complete and incomplete proteins:

FOOD	SERVING SIZE	PROTEIN CONTENT
Meat, fish, poultry*	4 ounces	28 grams
Eggs*	1 egg	7 grams
Cheese*	1 ounce	8 grams
Cottage cheese*	1/2 cup	16 grams
Milk, low-fat or whole*	1 cup	8 grams
Nuts	1 1/2 ounce	7 grams
Peanut butter	2 tbs.	7 grams
Soybeans	1 cup	23 grams
Dry beans and peas	1 1/2 cup	23 grams
Bean or pea soup	3/4 cup	7 grams
Bread	1 slice	3 grams
Dark green vegetables	1/2 cup	2 grams
Potatoes	1 medium	3 grams

*Complete proteins

To make incomplete proteins into complete proteins combine the following:

	EXAMPLE
Dried beans and peas with grains	Black beans and rice
Dried beans and peas with nuts or seeds	Garbanzo and sesame spread (hummus)
Grains with dairy	Macaroni and cheese
Grains with nuts	Peanut butter sandwich

Calcium: For Strong Bones and Teeth

Calcium is always important for women, but this is especially so during pregnancy. As your baby grows, it requires calcium to make its soft bones and teeth hard and sturdy. If you don't eat enough calcium, your body will take calcium from your bones and teeth to give to your baby. This could make your bones become brittle, weak, and thin and eventually cause osteoporosis. In addition, your teeth could soften, making them prone to cavities. Besides building strong bones and teeth, calcium is also necessary to control nerve impulses, keep your muscles working, and help clot your blood. Inadequate calcium can also result in high blood pressure, which during pregnancy can become a dangerous condition called preeclampsia. Obviously, now is the time to start eating more calcium.

Although most people know that dairy products are good sources of calcium, other nondairy foods may also be good sources. The following table lists some foods that all provide three hundred milligrams of calcium per serving. Remember, while you are pregnant you need twelve hundred milligrams of calcium per day, or about four choices from the following list (for example, four cups of milk per day).

CALCIUM SOURCE	SERVING SIZE
Whole milk	1 cup
Low-fat milk	1 cup
Skim milk	1 cup
Nonfat dry milk	1/3 cup
Plain yogurt	1 cup
Fruited/flavored yogurt	1 cup
Pudding	1 cup
Cottage cheese	2 cups
Ice cream	1 1/2 cups
Tofu	2 1/2 inches
Canned sardines (with bones)	2 ounces
Cooked dry beans	3 cups
Blackstrap molasses	2 tbs.
Cheese	1 1/2 ounces
Cooked broccoli	3 stalks
Cooked collard greens	1 cup

Getting enough calcium during pregnancy may be more difficult for those women who have trouble digesting dairy products, but it is certainly not impossible. Besides eating the nondairy calcium-rich foods listed above, such women may also try the following suggestions:

1. Drink *small amounts* of milk with meals, as combining milk with foods often makes it easier to tolerate.

2. Choose cheese, yogurt, or buttermilk, which are usually better tolerated.

3. Choose pudding, ice cream, frozen yogurt, or custard for calcium-rich desserts, which also seem to be better tolerated.

4. Eat foods made with small amounts of dairy products like tacos, pizza, and cream soups.

5. Select lactose-reduced milk (such as Lactaid or Dairy Ease).

You should also try to limit the amount of soft drinks you consume because soft drinks contain phosphates, which can reduce calcium absorption.

Pumping Iron

During pregnancy the volume of your blood nearly doubles because you develop extra blood vessels to feed and nourish your baby. Therefore, your need for iron, an important part of the blood, is increased. Iron is used by you and your baby to carry oxygen through your bloodstream. Your unborn baby needs to store enough iron during the nine months of pregnancy to help prevent anemia during its first six months of life since breast milk and non–iron-fortified formulas are poor sources of iron. Although many pediatricians prescribe iron-fortified formulas or pediatric liquid iron supplements, these do not replace your need for enough iron during pregnancy. Women of childbearing age need fifteen milligrams of iron. During pregnancy that requirement doubles to thirty milligrams, or three times what a man needs.

As with calcium, your baby will draw from your body's iron supply as he or she grows. This could leave you susceptible to anemia during and after pregnancy. Almost all health care providers recommend that in addition to an iron-rich diet, most pregnant women take a supplement containing at least thirty to sixty milligrams of iron per day. Be aware, however, that these high levels of iron may contribute to constipation. So to guard against this, try to increase your daily intake of fiber-rich foods and water.

Although an iron-rich diet is essential, not all foods containing iron are created equal. The iron in animal foods, such as lean red meats, is better absorbed and used by your body than the iron in spinach and other vegetables. Thirty percent of the iron in meat is absorbed, whereas only ten percent of the iron in vegetables is. To increase the amount of iron absorbed from vegetable sources, combine the vegetables with a vitamin-C-rich food such as orange juice or tomatoes. Better yet, combine a meat with an iron-rich vegetable to increase the amount of iron your body actually uses from the vegetable source. The following table provides information on the iron content of foods:

FOOD	SERVING SIZE	IRON CONTENT
Liver, beef, or poultry	3½ ounces	9 milligrams
Oysters	3½ ounces	8 milligrams
Kidney beans	1 cup	6 milligrams
Figs, dried	10	4 milligrams
Clams	½ cup	4 milligrams
Pork, chop or roast	3½ ounces	4 milligrams
Beef, steak or roast	3½ ounces	4 milligrams
Prune juice	1 cup	3 milligrams
Peas, split or green	1 cup	3 milligrams
Lamb, chop or leg	3½ ounces	3 milligrams
Blackstrap molasses	1 tbs.	2 milligrams
Raisins	⅔ cup	2 milligrams
Acorn squash	1 cup	2 milligrams
Shrimp, cooked	3½ ounces	2 milligrams

How to Increase Your Iron . . . Painlessly

1. Eat foods rich in Vitamin C such as citrus fruits, tomatoes, or broccoli to boost the absorption of iron from other foods. Also, take your prenatal vitamin containing iron with orange or grapefruit juice rather than water.

2. Don't drink coffee or tea with iron-rich foods or your prenatal vitamin. Both beverages decrease iron absorption.

3. Calcium blocks iron absorption. Never take your prenatal vitamin with milk or yogurt.

4. Cook in cast iron skillets or pots to add iron to food without changing the taste. Simmering spaghetti sauce or making vegetable soup in an iron pot can easily double the iron content of the meal.

5. Use only small amounts of water when boiling meats or vegetables. This will decrease the amount of iron lost in the cooking process. Then reuse the water in soups or stews.

6. Choose whole grain and iron-enriched breads, pasta, and other flour products. Processing often removes iron from the grain.

7. Eat red meat, fish, or poultry at least once a day. These animal foods contain easily absorbed iron.

A Note to Vegetarians

If you are a vegan vegetarian, meeting your protein, calcium, and iron needs through foods will be a challenge. For protein requirements you will need to make sure that you are eating adequate levels of complementary proteins. Not only will your calorie requirements be greater because you are pregnant, you will also have to eat a greater quantity of protein-rich plant foods. In terms of your calcium needs, you will want to focus on the nondairy calcium sources. A good option for you is to eat lots of tofu, which is a great source of protein and calcium. Since nonmeat sources of iron are poorly absorbed, you'll want to make sure you faithfully take your prenatal supplement in order to meet your iron needs. Also, focus on the tips for increasing your foods iron absorption and content.

Vital Vitamins

All vitamins are important during pregnancy. Highlighted here are three of the more well-known and important pregnancy vitamins.

Folic acid   Folic acid (also called folate or folacin) is one of the B vitamins. It works with protein and iron to build tissue and make extra blood for you and your unborn baby. During pregnancy your need for folic acid more than doubles to four hundred micrograms per day. It is so essential that your health care provider will almost certainly prescribe a folic acid supplement, which is included in all prenatal vitamins. Recently, the U.S. Public Health Service recommended that all women capable of becoming pregnant supplement their diets with four hundred micrograms of folic acid daily. This would reduce by half the risk of having a baby with a neural tube defect such as spina bifida (incomplete closure of the spinal cord) or anencephaly (no brain). Neural tube defects kill or disable nearly 2500 infants born in the

United States each year. In addition to your prescribed folate supplement, try to eat one to two cups of folate-rich foods daily. These include spinach, broccoli, collard greens, beets, cauliflower, brewer's yeast, legumes (such as split peas, soybeans, black-eyed peas, and chick peas), liver, avocado, melon, orange juice, and wheat germ. Don't overcook any of these, however, since folic acid is easily destroyed by long cooking.

Vitamin C   Vitamin C is essential for the development of bones, teeth, and blood vessels. It is also necessary for the formation of collagen, which in the body holds skin and bones together. If there is insufficient Vitamin C, your wounds would heal more slowly and abnormalities of your bones, gums, and teeth would occur. Vitamin C also helps the body increase the absorption of iron and convert folic acid to its active form. As mentioned before, both iron and folic acid are vitally important for pregnant women, therefore Vitamin C is too.

Your requirement for Vitamin C in pregnancy is seventy milligrams per day, or ten milligrams more than when you are not pregnant. This increased need can be filled easily by drinking just one cup of orange or grapefruit juice, eating one cup of broccoli, red or green peppers, brussels sprouts, cauliflower, strawberries, or cantaloupe. Treat your Vitamin-C-rich foods with care, however. Peeled or cut fruits and vegetables exposed to the air and all fruits and vegetables subjected to baking soda or excessive heat will have their Vitamin C destroyed. So don't overcook your vegetables, choose fresh rather than canned or cooked fruit, avoid canned fruit juice or vegetables (fresh or frozen is better), store your fruits and vegetables in airtight containers, and never add baking soda to improve the color of cooked vegetables.

Vitamin A   Vitamin A helps to develop special tissues in your growing baby including the outside covering of the eye (the cornea), and the linings of the digestive system, urinary tract, mouth, lungs, and sinuses. Vitamin A also helps with bone and tooth development, is necessary for night vision, and increases resistance to infections.

The RDA for Vitamin A is 4000 international units (IU) daily. There is no increased need for Vitamin A during pregnancy since it can be stored in your body. Although these reserve stores can potentially become depleted, you don't need Vitamin A on a daily basis. In fact, excessive amounts of preformed Vitamin A can cause birth defects in your unborn baby. The most dangerous time to take preformed Vitamin A is two weeks prior to conception and during the first two months of pregnancy. Too much preformed Vitamin A, even stored in the mother's body just before she becomes pregnant, can cause serious physical disabilities in an unborn baby. *Never* take a supplement of preformed Vitamin A unless it is prescribed by your doctor. This includes multivitamins with more than 10,000 IU per day.

The precurser to Vitamin A, called beta-carotene, is nontoxic and safe during pregnancy. It can be found in bright red, orange, yellow, or green fruits and vegetables. It's recommended that you eat several of these foods per week. Fruits and vegetables are your safest sources of Vitamin A.

Food sources of preformed Vitamin A include fortified milk, cheese, margarine, butter, and eggs. It is recommended that pregnant women or those considering becoming pregnant avoid liver, the richest food source of preformed Vitamin A, which contains 9000 IU in just three ounces. Try frequently to eat beta-carotene–rich fruits and vegetables such as squash, tomatoes, carrots, pumpkin, sweet potatoes, cantaloupe, papaya, apricots, peaches, spinach, turnip greens, and broccoli.

Nutritious Nibbles
Sometimes eating right during pregnancy can seem overwhelming. It may seem as if you have to eat so much food. One of the ways to make it easier for you to get all you need is to add small,

frequent nutrient-rich snacks to your daily diet. If you do this, you'll never have to eat large amounts of any food at any one time. That way, your stomach won't get overfull and you'll avoid feeling bloated and experience less heartburn, two common complaints during pregnancy. Also, isn't it fun to think that you can literally eat anytime? Snacks are really okay! Try these delicious and nutritious suggestions.

Sweet Snacks   Dried or fresh fruit; frozen, unsweetened fruit (eat partially thawed); apple slices with peanut butter; fig bars; applesauce; Teddy Grahams; granola bars; canned fruit in its own juice; graham crackers with fruit spreads; Frosted Mini-Wheats; pudding made with low-fat milk; fruited yogurt.

Crunchy Munchies   Shelled nuts or seeds; pretzels; popcorn (unbuttered); whole grain crackers; rice cakes; raw vegetables with yogurt dip; dry whole grain cereals; low-fat tortilla chips.

Hearty Helpings   Hard-boiled eggs; cheese slices; mozzarella sticks or cottage cheese; lean meat cubes; baked potato stuffed with broccoli and melted cheese; pizza bagels; peanut butter or lean lunch meat sandwiches; grilled cheese sandwiches.

Most of these snack foods are convenient to

carry with you. Remember, small snacks between meals can satisfy hunger, help prevent
nausea, and add vital nutrition to your diet.

Step Three: Appropriate Exercise

The amount of exercise that is appropriate during pregnancy largely depends on your prepregnancy level of fitness. You and your health
care provider should discuss the type and
amount of exercise that is right for you at the
different stages of pregnancy. Many women
find a combination program of low impact exercise like walking or yoga is beneficial when
alternated with a light-weight workout that
helps keep arms and upper body toned and
strong.

There are many reasons to work your pregnant body: 1) Exercise can prevent or ease
lower back pain, 2) Exercise can prepare you
for the demands of childbirth, 3) Exercise can
supply you with much-needed energy, and 4)
Keeping yourself fit during pregnancy can help
you get back into shape after the baby is born.
Most fitness experts recommend that pregnant
women should not exceed a heart rate of 140
beats per minute. To get a good workout you
should exercise hard enough to keep your pulse

at 120 beats per minute for ten to fifteen minutes (to check yourself, find your pulse at your neck and count the beats for ten seconds; then multiply by six). How much exercise is too much? The general rule is always be sure you are able to talk without gasping for breath at any time during your workout.

If you are planning an exercise program, keep in mind that the pregnancy hormones that allow your body to stretch to accommodate your growing baby also affect your ligaments and joints. It's easier, therefore, to overstretch certain parts of your body while you are pregnant. Because of this, gentle, low impact exercises such as walking, swimming, and cycling are preferred over jarring or bouncing activities such as running or high impact aerobics. Remember, if you choose an exercise plan that's right for you and your schedule, you're more likely to enjoy and stick with your pregnancy workout.

Although all women are different, the following advice for exercise during pregnancy is true for everyone:

1. Pregnancy is *not* the time to begin an intensive exercise program. The amount of exercise you got before pregnancy is probably okay during pregnancy as long as it doesn't lead to extreme exhaustion.

2. Moderate exercise is recommended, especially walking. Avoid long periods of strenuous exercise or short bursts of vigorous activity since hard exercise can raise your internal body temperature and can affect your growing baby. Be sure to warm up and cool down before and after all exercise.

3. Avoid skiing, mountain climbing, horseback riding, scuba diving, surfing, and other risky sports. Also, limit exercise in hot, humid weather or when you have a fever or don't feel well.

4. If you want to build or maintain muscle tone in your arms (for when you'll be carrying the baby around) try lifting three- to five-pound weights slowly, without straining.

5. Don't do deep-knee bends, full situps, double leg raises, or straight-leg toe touches.

6. Wear a well-fitting support bra.

7. Drink plenty of fluids before and after your workout.

8. *Always* consult your health care provider before starting an exercise program during pregnancy. For more information, you can ask your health care provider for a copy of the American

Academy of Obstetricians and Gynecologists
brochure *Exercise and Fitness: A Guide for
Women.*

Don't Overdo It!!
Immediately *Stop* exercise if you experience
any of these symptoms:

> bleeding
> abdominal cramping
> dizziness
> pubic pain
> back pain
> shortness of breath
> difficulty walking
> rapid heartbeat
> palpitations
> any unusual pain

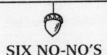

SIX NO-NO'S

Throughout your pregnancy, always remember
the following *critical* information necessary for
the delivery of a happy, healthy baby.

1. Alcohol: Stop drinking *now!* Alcohol causes
serious birth defects as well as mental and be-
havioral problems.

2. Drugs (prescription and over-the-counter): Be sure to tell your health care provider all the medicines you are taking. Many should not be taken during pregnancy.

3. Street drugs: Marijuana, cocaine, amphetamines (speed), and crack can deprive babies of oxygen and food. Babies can be born addicted to drugs or with birth defects. If you use so-called "recreational" drugs, stop now and get help. Treatment programs are available.

4. Cigarettes: Quit now! Nicotine constricts blood vessels so your baby gets less oxygen and nourishment. Smoking also increases the risk of miscarriage, premature birth, stillbirth, low birth weight, sudden infant death syndrome, and mental problems in newborns.

5. Caffeine: You don't need to avoid all caffeine, but discuss the use of coffee, tea, soft drinks, chocolate, and caffeine-containing over-the-counter medications with your health care provider.

6. Artificial sweeteners: Avoid saccharin since its effects on your unborn baby are not known; limit aspartame (Nutrasweet) to two servings per day, according to the American College of Obstetricians and Gynecologists' recommendation.

PREGNANCY, CHILDBIRTH, AND PARENTHOOD READING LIST

As you move through your pregnancy, there are a lot of books you can read to help clarify and enhance this magical time. You'll want to get started reading up on the basics of infant care and child rearing as well as what to expect while you're pregnant. The more you read now, the better prepared you'll be for the big day and the lifetime of love, laughter, and tears to follow. Here is a checklist of practical and inspirational titles.

What to Expect When You're Expecting by Arlene Eisenberg, Heidi Murkoff, and Sandee E. Hathaway, B.S.N. (Workman Publishing)

Infants and Mothers by T. Berry Brazelton, M.D. (Delta Books)

Guide to Baby Products by Sandy Jones with Werner Freitag and the Editors of Consumer Reports (Consumer Reports Books)

The Nursing Mother's Companion by Kathleen Huggins, R.N., M.S. (The Harvard Common Press)

Dr. Spock's Baby and Child Care by Benjamin Spock, M.D., and Michael B. Rothenberg, M.D. (Pocket Books paperback, E. P. Dutton Inc., hardcover)

Your Baby and Child by Penelope Leach, Ph.D. (Alfred A. Knopf)

On Becoming a Family by T. Berry Brazelton (Delta Books)

I Wish Someone Had Told Me: Comfort, Support, and Advice for New Moms from More Than 60 Real-life Mothers by Nina Barrett (Fireside Books)

Parents™ Book for Your Baby's First Year by Maja Bernath (Ballantine Books)

What to Expect the First Year by Arlene Eisenberg, Heidi Murkoff, and Sandee E. Hathaway, B.S.N. (Workman Publishing)

Section Three:
What to Do
the Second Trimester

As your second trimester begins, you will start feeling much more energetic. The extreme fatigue and nausea of the first trimester will fade away, leaving you feeling much like your old self. Now you'll actually begin to see and feel some changes in your body. By the third or fourth month people around you will also begin to notice something different. Perhaps it's that happy glow you're radiating or maybe it's the disappearance of your waistline and the bulge in your belly. Either way, it's a thrill when you first wear maternity clothes and your friends, coworkers, or complete strangers begin to treat you extra specially. Now that you do feel better, the second trimester is the time to do "housekeeping." You should register for and attend childbirth classes, check with your insurance company so you are up-to-date on your pregnancy coverage, go shopping for all your baby and maternity needs, and register for infant care classes often given at your hospital or through your childbirth education program.

TELLING THE BABY'S SIBLINGS

Your older child or children may or may not take the news of a new brother or sister in the way you'd hoped. To help promote the news as good news, introduce the idea in a happy, relaxed way. The following tips will help:

1. Wait until at least the second trimester to share the news. Nine months is a long time for any child to wait.

2. Tie your due date to an event that your child can understand, like "when the leaves fall from the trees" or "after your birthday."

3. Speak of the baby as "ours," not "mine."

4. Reassure your child that you'll always be there for him or her even though some things will be different after the baby. Remember to baby your first baby.

5. Increase the amount of special time you spend with your older child before the new baby arrives and especially after the birth.

6. If your hospital has one, sign your child up for sibling prep classes. Get him or her "I'm the big brother/sister" T-shirts and buttons. Read stories about new babies. Some educational and inspirational titles include:

Mommies Lap by Ruth Horowitz (Lothrop, Lee, and Shepard)

Big Like Me by Anna Grossnickle Hines (Greenwillow Books)

New Baby by Emily Arnold McCully (HarperCollins)

Waiting for Hannah by Marisabina Russo (Greenwillow Books)

The New Baby by Fred Rogers (Putnam)

New Baby at Your Home by Joanna Cole (William Morrow)

How You Were Born by Joanna Cole (William Morrow)

Getting Ready for New Baby by Harriet Ziefert (HarperCollins)

7. Ask your child to help decorate your hospital room and the baby's nursery. Help him or her make special pictures and crafts, or even homemade birth announcements.

8. If your hospital allows and your child is over two years, have your child come visit you. But make sure to prepare him or her for a hospital atmosphere first.

9. Include your firstborn in all the festivities surrounding the baby's birth. Word birth announcements using your child's name, such as "Rachel has a new sister."

10. Ask visitors to pay attention to your older child. Bringing a small gift for the older sibling along with a baby gift can help squelch negative behaviors and feelings.

11. Bring home a gift from the baby for the older sibling when you return from the hospital. A great gift is a baby doll that your child can take care of while you care for the new baby.

ANNOUNCING THE NEWS AT WORK

When sharing your happy news at work, plan your announcement carefully. As a rule of thumb, you should wait until the second trimester to inform your boss and coworkers of your pregnancy. By the third month your risk of early pregnancy loss is diminished, and telling people is easier and more joyful. Follow this checklist of steps when telling your boss about your pregnancy to safeguard your rights and help you successfully secure maternity (or paternity) leave.

Before the Announcement:

1. Get a performance evaluation. Even if it's not your usual review time, just tell your boss that you're interested in getting his or her opinion on how you're doing on the job. Afterward, request a memo from your boss confirming any feedback or promises. If you're unable to obtain a memo from your boss, you write the memo to your boss requesting a memo back if he or she disagrees with anything you've included. Be sure a copy goes into your employee record.

2. Find out as much as you can about your company's pregnancy and leave policies. Check with the human resources department, then ask other mothers how the company policy worked for them. When you give your boss the news, you will be negotiating from a knowledgeable standpoint. You don't want to seem like you're asking for a special favor. Be sure to ask about short-term or temporary disability benefits. If your company provides those benefits, you should be entitled to them.

3. Know your rights under the Family and Medical Leave Act. If your company has at least fifty employees, you've worked there at least one year, and you work twenty-five hours per week or more, you're entitled to twelve weeks of unpaid maternity leave. If you'd like to return to work gradually (e.g., part-time, working eventually back to full-time), you must first have your employers approval under the law. A growing number of companies allow new moms to ease back in to work after childbirth. A study conducted by the Families and Work Institute showed that employees who are given flexible schedules feel more loyal to their bosses, take greater initiative at work, and are more committed to helping their employers succeed. Explain this to your boss. He or she may not be familiar with this research.

When You Announce the News:

1. Tell your boss first. You want the news to come directly from you, not the grapevine.

2. Choose the right time. You'll probably begin to show during the second trimester of your pregnancy, so now is the time to bring up the subject. Try to catch your boss in a receptive mood, make an appointment, and never mention it nonchalantly when you don't have time to discuss its implications. For dads-to-be, put in for the leave as soon as you can. The more notice you give, the easier it will be for your boss and colleagues to prepare for your absence.

3. Be prepared to suggest dates for your departure and return.

4. Negotiate from a position of strength. Remind your boss of your skills and importance to the company, then ask how much time you can take. Remember, you're probably entitled to twelve weeks unpaid leave regardless of your company policy. If your boss is unresponsive or vague about your departure or return dates, remind him or her that you know your rights under the law and are prepared to fight for them. Make sure it is understood that taking maternity or paternity leave will not be used against you when it comes to promotions and assignments.

5. Confirm all details in writing. Take notes during all discussions, especially if you've negotiated changes in your schedule or responsibilities.

6. Be prepared to answer questions. Try to have a child care plan ready and be positive about the effects of new parenthood on your work life.

7. Watch out for subtle (and not so subtle) pregnancy discrimination. Know the law—the Federal Pregnancy Discrimination Act of 1978 makes it illegal for employers with more than

fifteen employees to fire, demote, or penalize
you in any way because you're pregnant. Some
states extend this law to companies with as few
as four employees. In spite of these protections,
however, pregnant workers may still be singled
out during layoffs. Pregnancy discrimination
includes any attempt by an employer to force a
woman to go on maternity leave before she is
willing or asking about pregnancy, child rearing, and/or child care during the hiring process. Common tactics include phasing out your
job during a downsizing or restructuring, only
to replace you with a new hire after you're
gone, or questioning your competence once
you announce your pregnancy.

If you believe you've been discriminated
against, immediately file a complaint with your
local Equal Employment Opportunity Commission (EEOC) office. Depending on the state in
which you live, you have 180 to 300 days from
the day you learn of the discrimination to register your complaint. Also see if your city has a
human rights commission. This agency handles
sex discrimination cases and may be willing to
investigate the case on your behalf. Check the
federal government listing in the phone book
for the EEOC and the local government listing
in the phone book for the human rights commission.

For more information on pregnancy discrimination and your rights, contact the

Women's Bureau Clearinghouse in the U.S. Department of Labor. Call 1(800)827-5335 to order a packet of information. Another free and confidential resource is the Nine to Five Job Problem Hotline at 1(800)522-0925. For additional information about your leave rights, send $4.95 to the Women's Legal Defense Fund, 1875 Connecticut Ave. N.W., Suite 710, Washington, D.C. 20009 and request *A Guide to the Family and Medical Leave Act: Questions and Answers.*

QUESTIONS ABOUT INSURANCE

Begin to acquaint yourself with your covered maternity benefits. Keep a list of everything that relates to pregnancy, prenatal care and delivery, and newborn care. Highlight issues that seem vague or could be misinterpreted so that you can speak with an insurance representative to get clarification. Most employers offer either private major medical and hospitalization insurance, called traditional indemnity plans, which allows you to choose your own health care provider, or a managed care plan such as a health maintenance organization (HMO) or Preferred Provider Organization (PPO), which allows you to choose only a health care provider affiliated with the specific HMO or PPO. With HMOs and PPOs you're usually covered for well-patient care such as routine prenatal visits, and well-baby care after delivery, as well as illness. HMOs and PPOs usually require a minimum copayment per visit, whereas private insurance requires you to meet a deductible before they will pay out any benefits.

Speak directly to your insurance company or the human resource specialist at work to answer these important questions:

✓ ✓ ✓ ✓ ✓ ✓ ✓ ✓ ✓ ✓ ✓ ✓ ✓ ✓ ✓

Insurance Questions Checklist

○ **1.** Is pregnancy covered? Some private insurance companies will pay for prenatal care and delivery only in women who develop life-threatening conditions or who require surgery such as an emergency C-section.

○ **2.** Do I have membership in an HMO, PPO, or major medical and hospitalization (private) coverage?

○ **3.** Is there a waiting period before my benefits take effect? Some plans won't cover any preexisting condition, so you must wait nine to twelve months before coverage for prenatal and postpartum care kicks in. If you become pregnant before the waiting period is over, you won't be eligible for any pregnancy benefits.

○ **4.** How much is my deductible or copayment? Is there a cap on total coverage?

○ **5.** What kind of preauthorizations are necessary? What must I do before getting care or entering the hospital? Most traditional and managed care plans require preauthorizations for almost all tests. Managed care plans also usually require a referral from your primary care physician to any specialist such as an obstetrician before care will be covered.

○ **6.** Do my maternity benefits cover a high-risk pregnancy, such as one in which diabetes is present, where the mother-to-be is of an age considered advanced for pregnancy, or where an incompetent cervix is involved? What about a cesarean delivery?

○ **7.** Does my policy restrict the type of room I can stay in?

○ **8.** What is the allowed length of stay in the hospital after delivery? What about coverage for an extended length of stay for myself or the baby?

○ **9.** Does my policy cover special lab tests, all medications, or at-home nursing? What services or conditions are specifically *not* covered?

○ **10.** Will my newborn be covered? Some insurance companies will automatically cover the baby for up to thirty days after delivery as a grace period until you can obtain full coverage. Some plans, however, require advance notice of the baby's arrival before any benefits for the baby will take effect. Find out how much notice they require, or you could be stuck with very large hospital nursery charges.

○ **11.** Will my premium increase with a new dependent? What forms will I need to add the baby to my policy? Try to gather these forms before the baby arrives.

○ **12.** How are claims submitted? Does payment go directly to my health care providers or to me?

○ **13.** Does my insurance pay for the services of a midwife or only for a physician?

○ **14.** Can part of the fee be paid for by my insurance and part by my husband's insurance?

○ **15.** Does my company offer a tax-deferred spending plan? This allows you to set aside a specific amount of money to pay for medical bills without being taxed on that money.

HEALTH CARE BUDGET FOR YOUR BABY

Keep track of all your baby health care–related expenses on the chart below:

	Estimated Cost	Actual Cost	Tax Deductible?
Health care provider Hospital Private room/Suite for husband sleep-in (check with hospital for availability) Special tests Medications/Prenatal vitamins			
Baby's hospital expenses Pediatrician's fee			
Childbirth preparation classes			
Child care			
Health insurance: For you For baby			

	Estimated Cost	Actual Cost	Tax Deductible?
Special prenatal classes: Infant care Nutrition Exercise Infant CPR			
Baby nurse or other household help			

YOUR MATERNITY WEAR

Expect to start wearing maternity clothes by the start of your second trimester. Although you can wear some of your regular clothes the first few months, now is the time when you need to concern yourself with proper fit and comfort. Usually, wearing larger sizes of nonmaternity clothing doesn't work. These clothes are typically too short to cover your growing belly, too wide in the shoulders, and too long in the sleeves and legs. The overall look can become frumpy. Of course exceptions do occur, so don't stop trying to find larger size nonmaternity bargains. As you begin to build your maternity wardrobe, look for versatility in items. Clothes that can be mixed and matched are the best, and *borrowed* clothes are even better. Your body has changed, but your taste in clothes has remained the same. You want to look your best—without spending a fortune. Maternity clothes can be outrageously expensive. It's easy to get caught up in the aura surrounding a maternity clothes store. You will get pampered (which is great!), but you may also leave the store with a huge dent in your budget. Try these tips for stretching your maternity wear budget and building a beautiful maternity wardrobe:

1. *Purchase quality lingerie.* This is not an area in which to scrimp. You'll need new bras to fit your larger breast size, cotton maternity underwear—choose from stretch cotton briefs, cotton bikini panties, or stretch cotton high-cut panties, and if you plan to breastfeed, nursing bras and nightgowns. You should wait until your third trimester to get the best fit on nursing wear. Give your back a break later in your pregnancy with a comfortable fitted camisole or belts with nonconstrictive bands that stretch across your abdomen and lower back. Three brands of special lingerie to help support your lower back, abdomen, and breasts include the Bellybra by Basic Comfort, the Prenatal Cradle, which can be obtained with a doctor's prescription and thus may be covered by insurance, and the Reenie Maternity Belt. Sometimes just wearing a leotard is enough support for your growing belly and breasts if they are not too heavy.

2. *Select basic pieces that are easy to wear and easy to match.* Skirts, jackets, pants, leggings, and jumpers should be interchangeable in your wardrobe. Tops and accessories can add the style and colors of your taste.

3. Since you'll be wearing the same maternity pieces over and over, *choose shades, colors, and patterns that are subtle* so you won't get tired of them by your seventh month!

4. Select *fabrics that can span two seasons.* Remember, you will be wearing these for about six months. As you choose, bear in mind that dark colors are slimming, while light colors in flowing fabrics will also flatter your growing figure.

5. Purchase *gentle support maternity stockings that match the color of your skirt* for a slimming look.

6. *A well-fitting basic pant* in a variety of colors is essential.

7. *Leggings are also a useful piece of clothing.* They can be used for exercise or under maternity tops, jackets, and tunics for a terrific casual look.

8. Try *boxed sets of four basic pieces*—a skirt, dress, tunic top, and leggings for winter or a tank, dress, shorts, and pants for summer. They come in basic black and/or white and are made from stretchy ninety percent cotton/ten percent spandex. The clothes can be worn together or with your other clothes. Check your local maternity shops or your baby magazines for more information.

9. *Check nonmaternity sources* like your husband's closet for comfy around-the-house items such as oversize tops and sweaters. Also consider men's drawstring pants and pajamas. Button-down fronts on oversize tops can later double as easy-access nursing wear.

10. *Try maternity resale shops* for great prices on gently used clothes.

11. *Borrow, borrow, borrow!!*

12. *Choose bolder, larger jewelry* than you would normally wear. This will help balance out your growing figure.

13. By the way, *your maternity size is usually your natural size.* If you wore a medium before pregnancy, you'll probably wear a maternity medium now.

✓ ✓ ✓ ✓ ✓ ✓ ✓ ✓ ✓ ✓ ✓ ✓ ✓ ✓ ✓ ✓
Maternity Wardrobe Checklist

FUNDAMENTALS	BOUGHT	BORROWED FROM
1 to 2 nightgowns or pajamas		
3 to 4 prenatal bras		
1 to 2 sleep bras (no underwire)		
3 to 4 maternity panty hose		
6 maternity panties		
1 maternity slip		

Remember, a light discharge is normal during pregnancy, so be sure to keep a supply of panty liners on hand to protect your undergarments and clothes.

CASUAL WEAR	BOUGHT	BORROWED FROM
2 to 3 comfortable stretch pants		
3 to 4 mix and match tops, including sweaters if you'll be pregnant in the winter		
1 jeans or denim skirt		

CASUAL WEAR	**BOUGHT**	**BORROWED FROM**
2 to 3 leggings or shorts		
1 to 2 coordinated separates		
1 to 2 flat shoes (possibly in a larger size, since your feet may grow during pregnancy)		
1 sneaker		
1 swimsuit and coverup		

CAREER WEAR	**BOUGHT**	**BORROWED FROM**
3 to 4 work dresses or jumpers		
2 to 3 shirts to match jumpers		
4 blouses		
1 to 2 pants		
1 to 2 flat shoes (possibly in a larger size since your feet may grow during pregnancy)		
1 cardigan or coat (nonmaternity swing coats work well during pregnancy)		
1 special occasion dress		

PLANNING AND EQUIPPING THE NURSERY (AND YOUR HOUSE TOO!)

Your baby's nursery is where he or she will begin and end each day, and spend time napping and playing at other times. It's important, therefore, to make it as comfortable and inviting as possible. But before purchasing anything, you'll want to take several things into consideration: safety, quality, versatility, space, and your budget.

Safety, Quality, and Versatility Check: Selecting Furniture and Equipment

Lots of decisions need to be made when creating a nursery, but none is more important than making this special room a safe place. Your baby's nursery (and the rest of your home) should be well equipped with durable and safe furniture and equipment. All baby products, whether new or used, should have protective covers over any part that might pinch (such as hinges) safety belts that fasten securely, and no sharp edges. All paints should be lead free, and all material should be washable and durable.

Plastic covers should be installed on all unused electrical outlets. Brand-new baby furniture is required by federal law to meet safety standards. In addition, look for the Juvenile Products Manufacturers Association seal on high chairs, strollers, playpens, and other items. The following checklist of current safety and quality guidelines and common sense buying tips should be used in determining your purchases whether you shop at an upscale baby furnishings store, a resale shop, or a yard sale. To get high quality, you'll want to spend more money on such essentials as a car seat, which will be used to keep your baby safe long into toddler- and childhood. Items that don't have safety concerns, such as your diaper bag or baby monitor, can be functional without being expensive. Put your money into what really counts: the safety of your baby. One more thing to consider, children quickly outgrow furniture designed for little people. To save money in the long run, try to purchase full-size items that will carry your baby and his or her belongings through the years.

The Essentials: Crib, Changing Table, Stroller, Car Seat, High Chair, Baby Monitor, Diaper Bag, Bouncy Seat

✓ ✓ ✓ ✓ ✓ ✓ ✓ ✓ ✓ ✓ ✓ ✓ ✓ ✓ ✓
Safety Checklist for Your Crib

○ **1.** All slats or spindles should be no more than 2³⁄₈ inches apart and none should be damaged in any way.

○ **2.** The mattress should fit snugly (no more than two fingers' width) against the crib sides.

○ **3.** The mattress support should be securely attached to head- and footboards.

○ **4.** Corner posts should be no higher than ¹⁄₁₆ inch to prevent entanglement of clothing or cords.

○ **5.** Make sure there are no dangerous cut-outs present in head- or footboards.

○ **6.** Drop side latches should hold sides securely and move easily with minimal noise.

○ **7.** Crib side should be able to be lowered with one hand and have a nontoxic plastic top piece for teething babies.

○ **8.** Choose a sturdy crib with a height-adjustable mattress support that can be lowered as your baby grows.

○ **9.** Consider a crib designed to turn into a toddler and twin bed. It might be more expensive, but you may actually save money in the long run. Cribs that convert only to toddler beds are not recommended, since they are often more expensive but don't have the long-term benefits of converting to a twin bed.

○ **10.** Don't scrimp on the crib mattress. A top of the line, firm, comfortable mattress is more important for your baby than all the fancy furniture or cute doodads on which you could spend your money.

○ **11.** If you place a mobile in the crib, consider these points: Try to see it from the baby's point of view. A good mobile design tilts the faces of the characters down so that your baby can easily see them. High contrast of black and white or even primary colors are easier for your baby to see than pastels. Remove mobiles once your baby can push up on her hands and knees.

SAFETY TIPS:

1. Do not place crib near blind or drapery cords. Your baby could become entangled and choke. Always secure cords away from baby's reach.

2. Do not use pillows in an infant's crib. They pose choking hazards.

3. Never use plastic bags to protect the crib mattress.

✓ ✓ ✓ ✓ ✓ ✓ ✓ ✓ ✓ ✓ ✓ ✓ ✓ ✓ ✓ ✓

Safety Checklist for Your Changing Table

○ **1.** Make sure your changing table comes equipped with a safety strap.

○ **2.** It should be large enough to accommodate a growing baby. You'll be using your changing table even when your tiny newborn becomes a robust, squirmy baby.

○ **3.** Choose one that has a diapering surface at a comfortable height for you.

○ **4.** If space is limited, consider a changing table that fits on top of the crib and flips down along the crib side when not in use.

○ **5.** Try using a chest of drawers with an attachable pad and safety straps or an attachable flip top instead of a standard changing table. The chest of drawers is more useful and versatile in the long run and the flip top is less expensive and can be attached to baby's dresser.

SAFETY TIPS:

1. Never leave your baby unattended on a changing table even if the safety strap is securely fastened.

2. Don't keep diapering accessories within your baby's reach. Depending on the style of changing table you're using, keep these items on a shelf or in a drawer.

✓ ✓ ✓ ✓ ✓ ✓ ✓ ✓ ✓ ✓ ✓ ✓ ✓ ✓ ✓
Safety Checklist for Your Stroller/Carriage

○ **1.** Make sure the seat belt and crotch straps are attached securely to the frame.

○ **2.** The seat belt fastener should be easy to lock but difficult for an older baby to unlock.

○ **3.** A wide canopy to block sun and light rain is an important feature.

○ **4.** It should have a wide base to prevent tipping.

○ **5.** The wheels should have locking brakes that set with the flip of a lever or press of a foot.

○ **6.** Wide or thickly padded wheels help make a smoother ride and textured wheels provide better traction on rough surfaces.

○ **7.** Removable and washable seat pads make cleaning much easier.

○ **8.** Umbrella strollers are great once your baby can be propped comfortably or sit on his or her own. They are smaller so they fit any-where and fold easily with one hand. Some of-fer fully padded reclining seats with good sup-port, but the more common hammock-style ones do not provide adequate support for newborns.

○ **9.** Height-adjustable handles are a comfort feature to consider.

○ **10.** Some strollers convert to a carriage by reversing the handle position. This type is a good choice, since it allows the stroller to grow with your baby.

○ **11.** Some carriages or strollers can also double as a bassinet.

SAFETY TIPS:

1. Don't hang bags from the handle of the stroller—it could tip over.

2. *Never* leave a child unattended in a stroller.

✓ ✓ ✓ ✓ ✓ ✓ ✓ ✓ ✓ ✓ ✓ ✓ ✓ ✓ ✓ ✓
Safety Checklist for Your Car Seat

❍ **1.** It should have at least a three-point harness system. Some car seats have a five-point harness system which secures the belt at the shoulders, crotch, and each hip. This is probably a feature that you want, since it means greater safety for your baby. Car seats with this feature may or may not cost more, depending on the brand.

❍ **2.** Make sure the seat is appropriate for your baby's weight and height. Babies under twenty pounds should ride in a rear-facing car seat. All car seats can be positioned in either a front or rear-facing position. Specially designed infant car seats, however, are the best for newborns and babies up to twenty pounds. See No. 3 for some money-saving ideas if you plan on using two car seats.

❍ **3.** Infant car seats are a convenience must. These car seats double as an infant carrier and can be clicked into and out of the car for maximum ease and comfort. Since you'll use this car seat for only a short time (about three to five months), try borrowing one from a friend or renting one from your local hospital (See No. 8).

○ **4.** Some available features such as reclining seats, swiveling seats, head rests, or storage space provide convenience. These extra options raise the price, however, and may not be worth the extra money.

○ **5.** Roll towels or a doughnut cushion prevent baby's head from flopping down while in the car seat.

○ **6.** You'll also want to get a baby shade for the car to block the sun.

○ **7.** Read the manufacturer's installation instructions carefully. Always make sure the seat is facing the proper direction and is attached to the car's safety belt correctly.

○ **8.** To save money, consider using a loaner or rental car seat. Programs that lend or rent car seats for a nominal fee are usually sponsored by hospitals and childbirth education associations. Also, ask your pediatrician or state highway safety department. They may be able to help you find a loaner program. Another low-cost

option is to purchase your car seat from Midas
Muffler. They offer low-cost car seats through
their Project Safe Baby™. You pay $42 for the
car seat, save the paperwork, and when the seat
is no longer needed, you return it to Midas and
receive $42 worth of free service. There is no
time limit on return of the car seat.

SAFETY TIP: Always strap baby into his or
her car seat, no matter how short the drive.

✓ ✓ ✓ ✓ ✓ ✓ ✓ ✓ ✓ ✓ ✓ ✓ ✓ ✓ ✓ ✓
Safety Checklist for Your High Chair

○ **1.** Make sure the high chair has waist and
crotch straps. These straps should be separate
from the tray and easy to lock and unlock.

○ **2.** The tray should lock securely.

○ **3.** The high chair should have a wide base
for stability.

○ **4.** Check to be sure that caps or plugs on
tubing cannot be pulled off and swallowed.

○ **5.** A folding high chair should have a secure
locking device to prevent collapse.

○ **6.** Several companies now have high chairs
that offer versatility and a good value. They

each are adjustable to six different height positions, so the chair can convert from an infant recliner to a high chair, and then to a toddler chair.

○ **7.** You can move a baby to a high chair as soon as he or she can sit with support, around five to seven months of age. Roll towels at the sides, back, and around baby's waist to help him or her fit more snugly in the beginning.

SAFETY TIP:

1. Place the high chair away from tables, counters, and walls so your baby can't push off them and topple.

✓ ✓ ✓ ✓ ✓ ✓ ✓ ✓ ✓ ✓ ✓ ✓ ✓ ✓ ✓ ✓ ✓
Safety and Convenience Checklist for Your Baby Monitor

○ **1.** Any baby monitor should be static free and give a clear sound indication when your baby is stirring. Be careful of portable telephones which can interfere with the use of your baby monitor. Check out various models in your home before the baby comes to see which one works for you.

○ **2.** Models with flashing lights as well as sound indicators are nice if you have a hearing problem or if you're watching TV, listening to the stereo, or vacuuming.

○ 3. Other features that you might want to include are a clip on receiver so that you can have the monitor with you in or outdoors, and/or a night light built into the base of the transmitter.

✓ ✓ ✓ ✓ ✓ ✓ ✓ ✓ ✓ ✓ ✓ ✓ ✓ ✓ ✓

Safety and Convenience Checklist for Your Diaper Bag

○ 1. Pockets, pockets, pockets! Outside pockets are convenient for carrying bottles, rattles, and other toys, or anything you'll need to get to quickly. Inside pockets will separate your wallet and keys from wipes and diapers. A special soiled diaper or clothes bag is a handy and sanitary option.

○ 2. Make sure it has a changing pad for easy diaper changes anywhere.

○ 3. Check for sturdy construction so that it will last you through your child's toddlerhood.

○ 4. An additional smaller diaper bag is nice for quick outings.

○ 5. A well-stocked diaper bag includes the following: diapers for newborns—you'll need *at least* six. Older babies require one for every hour you'll be out. Wipes—travel packs, travel-size diaper rash ointment, powder, and other diaper-change needs; two or three cloth diapers for spit ups and spills; a change of clothes; a plastic bag for wet, soiled items; a jacket or sweater; rattles and other toys; a front carrier; nursing pads if you are breast-feeding; bottles of formula or juice; any medicines such as acetaminophen; baby food, spoons, and a bib for older babies.

✓ ✓ ✓ ✓ ✓ ✓ ✓ ✓ ✓ ✓ ✓ ✓ ✓ ✓ ✓ ✓

Safety Checklist for Your Bouncy Seat

Bouncy seats are wonderful inventions every new mother should have. They allow your baby to be with you at all times: in the bathroom while you take a shower, in the kitchen while you prepare dinner, or in the yard while you garden.

❍ **1.** All bouncy seats should have a safety strap that is used at all times.

❍ **2.** Nice features on some include a detachable toy bar and a removable canopy for sun protection.

SAFETY TIP: Never place your bouncy seat on a high surface (countertop, table, etc.) once your baby can lift his or her head. Your baby could get up enough momentum to flip right off the surface, bouncy seat and all.

The Extras: Bathtub, Baby Swing, Playpen, Humidifier, Bassinet

✓ ✓ ✓ ✓ ✓ ✓ ✓ ✓ ✓ ✓ ✓ ✓ ✓ ✓ ✓ ✓ ✓
Safety Checklist for Your Baby Bathtub

❍ **1.** Be sure any baby bathtub you choose is either contoured for baby's body or cushioned to support baby's back, head, and neck.

❍ **2.** If you decide not to purchase a tub designed specifically for a baby, use sponge inserts to prevent slipping in the kitchen sink or family bathtub.

❍ **3.** If you're using a family bathtub, place a cover over the water spout and drain opener to protect your baby's head.

❍ **4.** Lower the temperature of your hot water heater to 120 degrees F to prevent burns.

❍ **5.** When you bathe baby, make sure the room is warm (around 75 degrees F) and free of drafts.

○ **6.** Sponge baths are best for newborns until the cord stump heals. Cradle the baby's head and neck with your arm to keep him or her secure in the tub.

○ **7.** You can move your baby from the infant tub to a bath ring anchored in the family tub once he or she can sit unassisted. Try placing a towel on the ring seat for fewer slips.

SAFETY TIPS:

1. Never leave a baby of any age alone in the tub, no matter where he or she is being bathed.

2. Keep all bathing accessories out of baby's reach.

✓ ✓ ✓ ✓ ✓ ✓ ✓ ✓ ✓ ✓ ✓ ✓ ✓ ✓ ✓
Safety Checklist for Your Baby Swing

○ **1.** Make sure the swing has a wide base to avoid tipping over.

○ **2.** It should also have secure straps that are easily fastened, and adjustable speeds.

○ **3.** Be sure the seat tilts back so the baby doesn't flop forward.

○ **4.** Newer models have no overhead piece, which makes getting baby in and out much easier and safer.

○ **5.** Quiet windup or battery-operated swings are preferred over hand-crank types, which could wake a sleeping baby.

SAFETY TIPS:

1. Always secure seat belt.

2. Never leave a baby unattended in a swing.

✓ ✓ ✓ ✓ ✓ ✓ ✓ ✓ ✓ ✓ ✓ ✓ ✓ ✓ ✓

Safety Checklist for Your Playpen

○ **1.** Wooden playpen should have slats or spindles no more than $2\frac{3}{8}$ inches apart.

○ **2.** Mesh playpens should have a small weave, no more than $\frac{1}{4}$-inch openings. Buttons and other decorations on a child's clothing could become caught on larger weaves, resulting in strangulation.

○ **3.** The mesh should have no tears, loose threads, or holes, and should be securely attached to the top and bottom rails. Torn mesh can pose a hazard for teething babies, who may bite off a piece and choke.

○ **4.** If the playpen has staples, all should be firmly in place with none missing or loose.

○ **5.** Portable play yards can double as a playpen or travel crib. They fold up quickly to the size of a large duffel bag and fit into a convenient carrying case for travel anywhere. Some have retractable canopies and/or roll-down flaps to help block wind and sun for use outdoors.

SAFETY TIP: Never leave a mesh playpen drop side down while the baby is in it. The area between the mattress and loose mesh can trap or suffocate a baby who rolls into that space.

✓ ✓ ✓ ✓ ✓ ✓ ✓ ✓ ✓ ✓ ✓ ✓ ✓ ✓ ✓ ✓
Safety Checklist for Your Vaporizer or Humidifier

Keeping the air in your baby's room humidified with a vaporizer or humidifier can help prevent upper respiratory infections and keep his or her delicate nasal passageways moist and healthy.

○ **1.** Steam vaporizer: use caution, as scalding is always a hazard when boiling water is present.

○ **2.** Warm mist humidifier: these units heat water and release the resulting steam. Like steam vaporizers, they pose a small scalding risk.

○ **3.** Cool mist humidifier: the American Academy of Pediatrics recommends cool mist units over steam vaporizers because they are just as effective but pose no danger.

○ **4.** Evaporative humidifier: no boiling water involved, units regulate mist output to keep air moist, not muggy.

SAFETY TIP: Whichever unit you decide to purchase, cleanliness is essential. Bacteria breed in standing water, so be sure to rinse, dry, and refill the unit daily. Once or twice a week the tank should be scrubbed out and thoroughly rinsed.

✓ ✓ ✓ ✓ ✓ ✓ ✓ ✓ ✓ ✓ ✓ ✓ ✓ ✓ ✓ ✓
Safety Checklist for Your Bassinet or Cradle

Both a bassinet or cradle are handy but not necessary during your baby's first few months. Some cradles have a rocking motion, which may lull your baby to sleep before he or she is able to be propped in a swing. If you choose a bassinet, remember, a bassinet should be lightweight and on wheels so it can be moved from room to room. (Some carriages can double as a bassinet.)

SAFETY TIP: The American Academy of Pediatrics recommends giving up the bassinet when your baby weighs ten pounds or is one month old. Some parents wait, however, until middle-of-the-night feedings are over before they move baby to a crib in the nursery.

For free baby safety information, write for the following pamphlets: *The Safe Nursery* and *Tips for Your Baby's Safety* available from the Consumer Product Safety Commission, Office of Information and Public Affairs, Washington, D.C. 20207. *Safe and Sound for Baby* available from Juvenile Products Manufacturers Association, 236 Route 38 West, Suite 100, Moorestown, N.J. 08057.

To check about recalled baby items, call:
U.S. Consumer Product Safety Commission 1(800)638-2772
National Highway Traffic Safety Administration 1(800)424-9393

Space in the Nursery

Before planning any decorating, be sure to examine your space. Now that you know which items are the essentials and which are the extras, you can begin the fun job of decorating. Think about what can optimize the area, both in terms of function and beauty. Window treatments should be functional. A sunny room may need room-darkening shades or curtains to help baby nap. This doesn't mean the shades and/or valences can't be beautiful, however. Try to color-coordinate the window coverings with the bedding. Some crib bedding sets actually come with a matching valence or curtains.

Wall space can help stimulate baby's visual senses, so consider pictures, mirrors, and wall coverings. Adding a border to a painted room is a less expensive alternative to wallpapering. It's also cheaper and easier to change a border than to scrape off wallpaper as your baby gets older and no longer wants teddy bears or baby jungle animals. Another inexpensive option for wall coverings are self-adhesive character sets. These are easy to put on and peel off and can be changed according to your child's whims.

The floor should be soft but durable and washable. If you have hardwood floors, consider a large nonskid rug, carpet tiles with a nonskid pad, or rubber mats. Carpeted floors are best, but try using rubber mats to protect messy play areas.

How to Measure the Room

1. Scale in a diagram of the floor plan.

2. Include measurements for windows, doors, closets, floors, any unusual corners, and their distance from each other.

3. Windows should be measured from inside the frame for blinds or shades, outside the frame for curtains.

4. To determine the amount of paint or wallpaper you will need, measure the wall area (ceiling height multiplied by wall length).

5. After determining the nursery dimensions, pencil in where each piece of furniture will go.

6. Carry the room measurements and scale drawings with you on your shopping trips.

Remember, Before Buying Any Item Ask Yourself These Questions: Could this tip over? Does it have sharp edges? Could my baby crawl into it and get stuck? Could it break into small pieces? Could my baby suffocate or choke? Is there any risk of strangulation?

✓ ✓ ✓ ✓ ✓ ✓ ✓ ✓ ✓ ✓ ✓ ✓ ✓ ✓ ✓

A Checklist Guide to the Basics for Lighting

○ **1.** If you can, avoid having the typical over-head light as the only light in the room. This will be too bright for baby's tender eyes, especially during middle-of-the-night diaper changes and feedings.

○ **2.** Try to use track lighting or a multilight fixture that can be directed where you need it.

○ **3.** Dimmer switches are helpful.

○ **4.** Although nursery lamps are cute, they outgrow their usefulness as your baby grows and redecorating becomes necessary. Purchase lamps that can grow with your baby's evolving taste.

○ **5.** Avoid freestanding lamps unless they are in a corner behind furniture. Your crawling baby can knock over an accessible freestanding lamp.

○ **6.** A night-light is essential. Choose one that automatically turns on as the room darkens. It'll be one less thing for you to remember to do at bedtime!

✓ ✓ ✓ ✓ ✓ ✓ ✓ ✓ ✓ ✓ ✓ ✓ ✓ ✓ ✓ ✓ ✓

A Checklist Guide to the Basics
for Storage Space

○ 1. Cubbyhole storage can organize clothing and toys.

○ 2. Vary the depth and height of shelves to accommodate different-size items.

○ 3. Avoid buying a deep-drawered dresser, which will lead to a mess when the entire contents are emptied to find the toy or piece of clothing on the bottom.

○ 4. Check out your nearest office supply store. Office equipment often comes with safety features such as a device to prevent file and other storage cabinets from tipping over. These items can be useful for safely storing your baby's belongings, especially when he or she begins to pull up on furniture.

○ 5. Try wire, molded plastic, or wicker baskets, or colored cardboard boxes to store books, lotions, small toys, rattles, and even diapers.

○ 6. Try a "toy hammock," which is specially designed to hold stuffed animals and other lightweight items. It's inexpensive and sold in toy or baby specialty stores.

○ **7.** Of course shelves work great for toys, books, and knickknacks. A more expensive alternative is a hutch that attaches to baby's dresser.

○ **8.** Use under-bed storage boxes for extra, out of season clothing or blankets. Store baby's toys in rolling bins under the crib.

○ **9.** If you use a toy chest, make sure hinges on the lid have support locks that hold it open, or better yet, choose one with a removable lid. Also, make sure that the chest has ventilation holes and that they will not be blocked if the chest is placed against a wall.

Nursery Plans

Theme:

Bedding pattern:

Color scheme:

Window measurements:

Room dimensions:

✓ ✓ ✓ ✓ ✓ ✓ ✓ ✓ ✓ ✓ ✓ ✓ ✓ ✓ ✓
Nursery Furniture Checklist

ITEM	BOUGHT	BORROWED FROM
bassinet or cradle		
crib and mattress		
changing table and pad		
dresser or chest of drawers		
rocking chair or glider		

✓ ✓ ✓ ✓ ✓ ✓ ✓ ✓ ✓ ✓ ✓ ✓ ✓ ✓ ✓
Nursery Accessories Checklist

ITEM	BOUGHT	BORROWED FROM
laundry hamper		
crib mobile		
nursery monitor		
nursery lamp		
crib mirror/black and white face		

ITEM	BOUGHT	BORROWED FROM
diaper bag		
baby bath		
infant carrier		
diaper stacker		
cloth diapers (for your shoulder)		
portable seat (for restaurants)		

✓ ✓ ✓ ✓ ✓ ✓ ✓ ✓ ✓ ✓ ✓ ✓ ✓ ✓ ✓ ✓ ✓ ✓ ✓

Nursery Bedding Checklist

ITEM	BOUGHT	BORROWED FROM
3 bassinet/cradle sheets		
3 fitted crib sheets		
1 quilted, waterproof crib pad		
2 to 3 crib blankets		
1 comforter or quilt		
crib bumpers		
crib ruffle		

Buying for Baby:
The Best-Dressed Newborn

The right wardrobe can make those first few months after birth easier on parents and baby. Many parents-to-be, however, go "oh-so-cute" crazy and end up purchasing the most adorable but also the most expensive and impractical items they see. Newborn and infant clothes should be comfortable for baby and convenient for Mom and Dad to put on and take off. Once you know what to look for and what to avoid, dressing your baby can be fun and easy. Use the following guide to universal baby-friendly features for all your infant clothes purchases: *easy access* to diaper area, *smooth seams* to avoid irritation to baby's delicate skin, *snug cuffs* to keep out cold air in winter or air-conditioning in summer, and *built-in feet* to prevent pants from riding up and to keep feet covered since booties and socks often fall off. If you receive gifts that do not meet these standards, return them or exchange them for more appropriate items. Here's a checklist of helpful tips for outfitting your new baby:

✓ ✓ ✓ ✓ ✓ ✓ ✓ ✓ ✓ ✓ ✓ ✓ ✓ ✓ ✓
Baby Clothes Purchasing Checklist

❍ **1.** Avoid purchasing clothes with drawstrings, as they pose a choking hazard.

❍ **2.** In the first few weeks, be gentle with fragile neck muscles by opting for side-snap or side-tie T-shirts. As your baby grows, add T-shirts with a wide opening at the neck so that they can easily slip over his or her head.

Onesies are the best, since they have crotch snaps and will stay tucked.

○ **3.** Go easy when buying newborn-to-three-month sizes, or better yet, skip them altogether. Your baby will outgrow these things very fast. Begin purchasing items in size six months except for the one outfit your baby wears home from the hospital. If you receive lots of newborn-to-three-month sizes as gifts, return them or exchange them for larger sizes.

○ **4.** When choosing a size, use your baby's weight and length rather than age as your guide.

○ **5.** Always look for crotch zippers, crotch snaps, or neck-to-toe zippers. Never buy baby clothes that don't have a way to get to the diaper without completely undressing the baby!

○ **6.** Avoid clothes that button or snap down the back, these are a real hassle.

○ **7.** Avoid Velcro closures, which invariably don't work after several washings.

○ **8.** Look for fabrics that are machine washable and do not require ironing. Clothes that are made of at least part cotton are extra soft and comfortable.

○ **9.** Decorations can poke an infant in uncomfortable places.

○ **10.** When you shop for sleepwear, look for a label that tells you it meets federal safety regulations and is flame retardant.

○ **11.** How much to buy depends on the following:

    a. Your access to a washer and dryer
    b. Whether you use cloth or disposable diapers (cloth diapers leak a bit more)
    c. How often your baby spits up

TIP: To determine if your baby is warm enough, use your own body temperature as a guide, then add a layer for your baby.

✓ ✓ ✓ ✓ ✓ ✓ ✓ ✓ ✓ ✓ ✓ ✓ ✓ ✓ ✓ ✓
Layette Checklist

The newborn layette is a list of clothing essentials for your new baby. The tiny items listed will be used by your baby for about the first three months of his or her life. They should be selected with care, always keeping safety concerns in mind. Although the new vocabulary and terminology of the layette may seem confusing at first, you'll soon become an expert at differentiating among kimonos, stretchies, and onesies! The following checklist should help you with your purchasing decisions:

BABY CLOTHES	BOUGHT	BORROWED FROM
4 to 6 side-snap or tie T-shirts		
4 to 6 slip-on T-shirts		
4 to 6 onesies (baby bodysuit)		
3 to 4 one-piece stretchies (one-piece coveralls)		
1 to 2 gowns, kimonos (remember, *no* drawstrings)		
2 to 4 booties/socks		
2 to 4 bibs		
3 to 4 sleepers (these are stretchies especially designed to be used as sleepwear)		
2 to 3 blanket sleepers (for winter)		
sweater or jacket		
brimmed hat/bonnet/hat with earflaps (depending on the season)		
snowsuit/bunting (if needed)		
2 sunsuits (if needed)		

BATH AND TOILETRY
3 to 4 hooded towels
3 to 4 washcloths
baby soap
baby shampoo
baby lotion
brush and comb
digital baby thermometer (rectal, ear, or oral; for axillary temperature)
baby scissors or nail clippers
alcohol pads until the umbilical stump falls off
petroleum jelly or A and D ointment

Diapering Choices: Some Helpful Hints

As your baby's due date approaches, you may be considering the different diapering alternatives available: home-washed cotton diapers, a diaper service, or disposable diapers. When making your decision, consider the following:

✓ ✓ ✓ ✓ ✓ ✓ ✓ ✓ ✓ ✓ ✓ ✓ ✓ ✓ ✓
Checklist of Diapering Questions

○ **1.** Which method will keep my baby most comfortable?

○ **2.** What will it cost over 24 to 36 months of daily diaper changes?

○ **3.** Which is most convenient for my life-style?

○ **4.** Do I have a washer and dryer? Is a laundromat convenient and clean?

○ **5.** What are the environmental consequences of each method?

○ **6.** Which type of diaper is the least leaky? (Disposable diapers have been found to leak less than cloth diapers.)

○ **7.** How do I feel about using pins? Can cloth diapers be used without pins?

○ **8.** Is my child's caregiver familiar with using cloth and/or disposable diapers?

After selecting a diapering method, consider the following list of helpful hints for diapering your baby:

1. Change a newborn frequently, ten to twelve times a day. As your baby grows older, fewer changes are needed.

2. Clean and dry your baby's bottom completely at changing time. Disposable baby wipes or a soft cloth with mild soap and water are acceptable. Always dry thoroughly with a soft towel or cloth before putting on a fresh diaper.

3. Use lotions or powders—never both at the same time. You'll end up with a sticky, dough-like paste. Try using pure cornstarch, which is nonirritating, or a zinc oxide ointment to help prevent diaper rash.

4. Air out your baby's bottom for several short periods during the day. The air will also help prevent diaper rash.

5. Consider having a diaper pail on each level of your home. This reduces trips up and down stairs to change and dispose of dirty diapers. Buy a diaper pail with inside flaps to help keep odors from escaping. For disposable diapers, you also might want to try a Diaper Genie, which is a specially designed diaper pail that eliminates disposable diaper odor by individually sealing each diaper. The Diaper Genie is more expensive than a standard diaper pail but may be worth it if you plan to keep a diaper pail in your family's living space.

Whichever method of diapering you choose, use the following checklist to make sure you have enough diapers on hand at home to get you through your first week. If needed, you can always send Dad out to buy more cloth or disposable diapers after that, or speak to your diaper service about increasing your weekly order.

✓ ✓ ✓ ✓ ✓ ✓ ✓ ✓ ✓ ✓ ✓ ✓ ✓ ✓ ✓ ✓
Initial Diaper Supply Checklist

DIAPER SERVICE: Contract them 2 weeks before your due date and order 80 to 100 diapers the first week.
HOME-WASHED DIAPERS: Purchase 3 to 4 dozen plus 4 diaper covers for your start-up supply.
DISPOSABLE DIAPERS: Purchase at least 1 bag of 50 newborn-size diapers initially.

✓ ✓ ✓ ✓ ✓ ✓ ✓ ✓ ✓ ✓ ✓ ✓ ✓ ✓ ✓ ✓
Diapering Checklist

cotton balls
diaper rash ointment
premoistened wipes
non-talc baby powder or pure cornstarch
A and D ointment or petroleum jelly
diaper covers (for cloth diapers)
diaper pail

A Word About Laundry

1. If you don't have a washer and dryer, now is a good time to invest in a pair. You'll be making lots of trips to the laundry room (or Laundro-mat) after your baby arrives.

2. Wash all your baby's clothes before wearing, even brand-new, unworn items. Fabric finishes on new clothing can be irritating to baby's tender skin.

3. Wash your baby's clothes separately in warm water with a mild detergent, *not* soap. Even soaps designed especially for washing baby clothes can remove the flame-retardant properties on children's sleepwear.

4. Keep chlorine bleach, color-safe bleach, and other stain removers on hand.

5. Always wash cloth diapers separately.

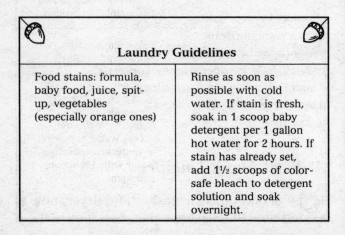

Laundry Guidelines

| Food stains: formula, baby food, juice, spit-up, vegetables (especially orange ones) | Rinse as soon as possible with cold water. If stain is fresh, soak in 1 scoop baby detergent per 1 gallon hot water for 2 hours. If stain has already set, add 1½ scoops of color-safe bleach to detergent solution and soak overnight. |

Laundry Guidelines

Oily, greasy stains	Pretreat with liquid laundry detergent and wash as usual, using the hottest temperature safe for the garment.
Mildew	Use chlorine bleach if safe for the fabric. If not, presoak in baby detergent solution and then launder. Prevent mildew: do not leave damp clothes in a hamper.
Other stains	Presoak in color-safe bleach, use liquid stain removers and/or liquid detergents generously.
Diaper soils (if you don't use a diaper service or disposable diapers)	Rinse diapers with cold water immediately. Presoak in baby detergent solution plus ½ cup color-safe bleach for minimum 30 minutes. Wring out excess water and wash in hottest temperature water with 1½ scoops detergent.

Choosing the Right Childbirth Class

Nearly all expectant parents attend childbirth classes. First-time parents usually start classes in their sixth or seventh month but start their search earlier to assure their place in class. Many childbirth classes have a long waiting list. You'll want to find a class that suits your needs in terms of type, length, cost, and location. Studies of women who attend these classes show that they generally require less medication, have fewer forceps deliveries, and frequently feel more positive about their birthing experience than women who do not take classes. All childbirth classes offer certain basics: emotional support, information on labor and delivery including both vaginal and cesarean births, techniques for muscular control and relaxation during labor, education about hospital procedures, and practice for expectant couples to work as a team during labor, delivery, and the postpartum period.

All classes are not alike, however. There are three major childbirth groups that certify instructors to teach their basic childbirth philosophies: ASPO (American Society for Psychoorophylaxis in Obstetrics)/Lamaze, the American Academy of Husband-coached Childbirth for the Bradley Method, and ICEA (International Childbirth Education Association).

ASPO/Lamaze

This program emphasizes active concentration based on relaxation. It helps to condition mothers-to-be through continuous training using patterned breathing techniques to replace unproductive laboring efforts with ones that allow labor to progress. Usually Lamaze classes run for five to six weeks toward the end of your pregnancy for a total of about twelve hours.

The Bradley Method

This program emphasizes relaxation with an inward focus. Unlike Lamaze, the Bradley Method does not teach specific breathing patterns. Rather, it puts strong emphasis on deep abdominal breathing similar to breathing while asleep. The American Academy of Husband-coached Childbirth opposes medication during labor. Couples who enroll in Bradley classes have usually decided not to use medication during labor and delivery. Classes begin as soon as pregnancy is confirmed and consist of twelve two-hour sessions emphasizing nutrition, breastfeeding, and exercise.

ICEA

This program does not emphasize any particular method. It educates couples about childbirth alternatives including the risks and benefits of medications, and how to ask questions to make informed choices. Some programs do teach relaxation techniques with patterned breathing. Class length varies.

Resources for Locating
Local Instructors
ASPO/Lamaze
1200 19th St. N.W.
Suite 300
Washington, D.C. 20036
1(800)368-4404

American Academy of Husband-coached
    Childbirth (Bradley Method)
P.O. Box 5224
Sherman Oaks, CA 91413
1(800)423-2397

International Childbirth Education
   Association (ICEA)
P.O. Box 20048
Minneapolis, MN 55420
1(612)854-8660

Your health care provider/hospital

"Childbirth education" section of the
   yellow pages

Friends and family who have had babies

To determine which type of class is right for
you, see the following checklist.

✓ ✓ ✓ ✓ ✓ ✓ ✓ ✓ ✓ ✓ ✓ ✓ ✓ ✓ ✓ ✓ ✓
**Checklist of Questions for
Childbirth Classes**

○ **1.** How much time do I want to spend on
childbirth classes?

○ **2.** How much money do I want to spend on
childbirth classes?

○ **3.** Was this program recommended by my
health care provider?

○ **4.** Does this program share my philosophy
of childbirth? How about the philosophy of my
health care provider?

○ **5.** How important is it that I avoid medications or other interventions?

○ **6.** Does this program begin when I need it (by the seventh month of pregnancy)?

○ **7.** Does this program have a small class size?

○ **8.** Did other expectant couples learn what they needed to know in this program?

○ **9.** Is the information accurate, interesting, and up-to-date? (Request a course outline ahead of time.)

○ **10.** Will we be able to meet other expectant parents?

○ **11.** Does this program include opportunities to ask questions, practice helpful techniques, and talk to parents who recently gave birth?

Breast- or Bottle-Feeding

Once you have begun your classes, and as your body grows and changes, the baby's arrival will seem more imminent. Another of the many things you will need to make decisions about at this time is whether to breast- or bottle-feed your baby. As an expectant parent, this is one of the most important decisions you will make. The following checklists will help.

✓ ✓ ✓ ✓ ✓ ✓ ✓ ✓ ✓ ✓ ✓ ✓ ✓ ✓ ✓

Breast-Feeding "Things to Consider"

○ **1.** Breast milk is the best choice nutritionally for your baby. It has been found to contain over one hundred ingredients, many of which help protect your baby against allergies and illness.

○ **2.** Breast milk cannot be mixed improperly, served at the wrong temperature, or contaminated.

○ **3.** Breast milk is easily digested, but because of this babies need frequent feedings.

○ **4.** Breast milk can be frozen or refrigerated and fed by bottle. This can help a new mom and baby take more outings. Out-of-the-home nursing can also be done modestly and discreetly using nursing tops or small blankets, cloth diapers or towels to cover your breast. Only four states, however, have passed laws that protect a woman's right to breast-feed in public; New York, California, Florida, and Virginia.

○ **5.** Breast-fed babies rarely become obese.

○ **6.** Nursing helps you burn up fat deposits laid down during pregnancy.

○ **7.** Nursing provides close body contact for you and your baby.

○ **8.** Night feedings can be done in bed with little disturbance since your milk supply is always with you.

NOTES:

1. You do not need and should not use any special creams or lotions on your nipples. Also, it's not necessary to toughen up your nipples during pregnancy to prepare for breast-feeding. In fact, too much nipple stimulation may result in premature labor.

2. Many professionals are available to help with breast-feeding: La Leche League at 1(800)LA-LECHE; the Nursing Mothers Council at 1(408)272-1448; your health care provider, especially a midwife; or a lactation consultant. Check with your hospital to see if they have one on staff or check the yellow pages.

If you choose to breast-feed, you'll want to ensure that your baby is getting enough milk.

Use the following checklist to help you make
the determination.

✓ ✓ ✓ ✓ ✓ ✓ ✓ ✓ ✓ ✓ ✓ ✓ ✓ ✓
Breast-Feeding Adequacy Checklist

○ **1.** Your baby has at least six to eight wet
diapers every day.

○ **2.** Your baby has frequent bowel movements—after every nursing is common for
breast-fed babies.

○ **3.** Your breasts feel softer or less full after
feeding.

○ **4.** You can see or hear your baby sucking.

If you have any doubts, consult your pediatrician immediately.

✓ ✓ ✓ ✓ ✓ ✓ ✓ ✓ ✓ ✓ ✓ ✓ ✓ ✓
Breast-Feeding Equipment Checklist

○ **1.** *Good nursing bras* should be one hundred percent cotton, have flaps that easily open
with one hand, and have no underwires. You
should be able to expose one breast at a time.
For accurate sizing, wait until the end of your
third trimester to shop for nursing bras.

○ 2. *Nursing pads* are necessary between feedings to collect leaked milk. They come in two types: disposable or washable. All should be cotton and contoured for a comfortable fit.

○ 3. A manual, battery, or electric *breast pump* is an absolute must if you plan on bottle-feeding expressed breast milk. Manual pumps work best for moms who need to pump milk only occasionally. They are lightweight and some work just as well, if not better, than battery-operated pumps. Women who pump more often than once or twice a day, however, should try using a larger electric pump, which produces a pumping action most similar to a baby's sucking.

○ 4. You should have *access to a refrigerator or cooler*. Although breast milk may keep safely for up to ten hours at room temperature, chilling it as soon as possible ensures its safety. Refrigerated breast milk can keep for no more than forty-eight hours. Frozen breast milk can keep for up to six months.

○ 5. For feeding or storage, you'll need plenty of glass or plastic *bottles* or disposable plastic liners. Purchase bottles in four-ounce and eight-ounce sizes. You may express your milk into an eight-ounce bottle but switch to a four-ounce bottle for feeding.

○ **6.** You'll also need at least four to six *nipples*. There are three types of nipples that come in rubber or clear silicone—regular, short, or orthodontic. The jury is still out as to which nipple is the best. You should try all three types with your baby to see which kind he or she prefers.

○ **7.** For cleaning your bottles and nipples, you'll need a *bottle and nipple brush* for hand washing and a *dishwasher basket* or *nipple racks* for the dishwasher. If you do not have a dishwasher, you may also want to consider a *sterilizer.*

○ **8.** *Clothes designed for nursing* eliminate the need to get undressed each time you nurse or express milk. For a list of all the companies that make clothing for nursing mothers, send a self-addressed stamped envelope to: The Association for Breast-feeding Fashions, P.O. Box 4378, Sunland, CA 91041. Consider the following list of ideas for dressing while nursing:

    a. Wear tops with patterns—they're less likely to show stains.
    b. Carry a jacket or sweater as a coverup just in case of leaks.
    c. Keep a spare blouse at work or in your car.

✓ ✓ ✓ ✓ ✓ ✓ ✓ ✓ ✓ ✓ ✓ ✓ ✓ ✓ ✓
Bottle-Feeding "Things to Consider"

○ **1.** Formula takes longer to be digested so baby feels full longer. Feedings can be less frequent.

○ **2.** Bottle-feeding never causes you any discomfort.

○ **3.** A day's supply of formula can be mixed all at once to save time.

○ **4.** Anyone can bottle-feed your baby, freeing you up to do other things. Bottle-fed babies should still be held close at all feedings, however, to give them a sense of closeness and comfort.

○ **5.** You won't have to worry about exposing your breasts in public if you bottle-feed.

○ **6.** You won't need to buy special bras, breast pads, or breast-pumping devices.

○ **7.** Dad can help with night feedings, allowing you more needed rest.

○ **8.** It's usually easier to bottle-feed if you plan to return to work soon after having your baby.

○ **9.** Fluoridated tap water used to mix formula precludes the use of fluoride supplements. Also babies who drink iron-fortified formula do not require iron supplements.

○ **10.** You can choose from ready-to-feed, concentrated, or powdered formulas based on economy, your baby's preference, and convenience.

○ **11.** You never have to worry that your baby is not getting enough milk. With bottle feeding you can quantify the amount your baby drank.

✓ ✓ ✓ ✓ ✓ ✓ ✓ ✓ ✓ ✓ ✓ ✓ ✓ ✓ ✓ ✓
Bottle-Feeding Equipment Checklist

○ **1.** The correct type of *formula* as prescribed by your pediatrician. The form of the formula does not matter (e.g., whether the formula is a ready-to-feed, powder, or concentrate) but rather the ingredients of the formula (e.g., whether it's milk or soy based or iron fortified or low iron) is what counts. Purchase only a few cans at first to make sure your baby can tolerate it and won't need to switch to a different type. Also try to stick with one form of formula in the beginning. It can confuse a baby to change back and forth from a thin, powdered formula to a thicker ready-to-feed and vice versa.

○ **2.** Plenty of glass or plastic *bottles* or disposable plastic liners. Purchase bottles in four-ounce and eight-ounce sizes. You'll use the smaller-size bottles for at least the first three months when your baby will be taking only one to four ounces at a feeding.

○ **3.** At least four to six *nipples.* There are three types of nipples that come in rubber or clear silicone—regular, short, or orthodontic. The best type for your baby is the one he or she prefers. You can also purchase newborn-size nipples if the standard size is too large for your baby's mouth.

○ **4.** For cleaning your bottles and nipples, you'll need a *bottle and nipple brush* for hand washing and a *dishwasher basket* or *nipple racks* for the dishwasher. If you do not have a dishwasher, you may also want to consider a *sterilizer.*

○ **5.** A *drying rack* to allow cleaned bottles to air dry in a sanitary manner.

○ **6.** If your baby will drink only warm formula and you are using the ready-to feed type, you will probably need to purchase a *bottle warmer.* Try finding one that is portable and can be used in the car during long trips. If you use powdered or concentrated formula, you can make a warm bottle by using warm tap water. Test the temperature of the bottle using the tried and true method of shaking a few drops on your wrist. Never heat a bottle in the microwave. The uneven heating that results from microwave use can cause an isolated hot spot to burn your baby's mouth even though the bottle temperature seems right to you.

Finding the Right Balance: Breast- and Bottle-Feeding

Choosing to breast- and bottle-feed may give you the best of both worlds. If you must return to work, or if Dad wants to get involved with feedings too, switching back and forth from breast to bottle makes sense. Whenever possible, however, feed your baby expressed breast milk in a bottle rather than formula. The baby will get the health benefits of drinking breast milk and you will help keep your milk supply from drying up completely. If this is not possible, try to gradually reduce breast-feeding sessions to avoid engorgement or breast infections.

Dads Are Pregnant Too

Prefatherhood can be a lonely time for some expectant dads. While mothers develop a special bond with the growing baby for nine months, fathers-to-be can feel isolated and may need some help to become comfortable with the idea of fatherhood. Use the following to help your partner get involved and be the best dad he can be:

✓ ✓ ✓ ✓ ✓ ✓ ✓ ✓ ✓ ✓ ✓ ✓ ✓ ✓
Idea Checklist

❍ **1.** Encourage your partner to attend as many monthly prenatal appointments as possible. He should be there when you first hear the baby's heartbeat and if an ultrasound is performed.

❍ **2.** Get your partner to read all the pregnancy, childbirth, and parenthood books that you are reading. Discuss what you've learned. Also make sure he attends childbirth classes and tours the maternity unit with you.

❍ **3.** Encourage him to talk to other new or expectant fathers for information and support.

❍ **4.** Encourage your partner to become involved by pretending he is pregnant too. He should do everything you do: quit smoking or taking recreational drugs, eat properly, and exercise.

○ **5.** Encourage your partner to talk or sing to the baby in utero.

○ **6.** You should be a good listener, be supportive, and be appreciative. Allow your partner to talk about his fears, hopes, and expectations without being judgmental. Assure him that he'll be a huge help to you at birth by just being there.

○ **7.** Make a plan for sharing household responsibilities after the baby comes. Start with a list of chores each of you doesn't mind doing, then divide the other jobs up evenly. Don't forget about new-baby chores.

○ **8.** Encourage him to take as much time off from work as possible after the baby arrives. Leave him alone with his new son or daughter so they can get to know each other and encourage solo daddy-baby outings.

○ **9.** Agree to keep romance alive. Try to have a date at least one to two times per month after the baby is born. Remember, the best gift a father can give his child is to love its mother.

Traveling for Two

The second trimester is the safest time for you to travel. Although travel is generally safe at other times during pregnancy, the fourth through sixth months present the lowest chance of complications. The risk of miscarriage goes down after the first trimester, and other prenatal complications such as hypertension or toxemia usually haven't developed yet.

Whether you're traveling by car, plane, bus, or train, take these extra steps to help keep you safe and comfortable:

1. Get the okay from your health care provider. Make sure you tell him or her what mode of transportation you are planning to use. Certain transportation, like motorcycles, is not usually recommended during pregnancy. If you're planning a cruise, check with your travel agent for any pregnancy restrictions and keep in mind that if you've never been on a ship before, pregnancy is probably not a good time to start, since sea travel can cause severe stomach upset.

2. Always use a car seat belt. Riding in a car without wearing a seat belt increases the risk to both you and your baby in the event of an accident. Make sure the lap belt is positioned below your abdomen and try putting a soft towel or blanket between you and the belt for greater comfort.

3. If you are traveling by car, tuck a pillow behind the small of your back, recline your seat, prop up your feet, and wear loose-fitting clothes. Plan for frequent stops at rest areas to walk around and go to the bathroom and try not to drive more than five or six hours each day.

4. If you are traveling by plane, ask for an aisle seat so that you can walk around and get to the bathroom easily. Also, ask for a seat in the forward part of the cabin, in front of the wings, for the most stable ride. If you can, get a seat by the wall dividing first class and coach; you'll get extra leg room or, better yet, splurge for a first class ticket!

5. Remember that most airlines won't let women fly in their ninth month without written permission from their health care provider. Allow yourself plenty of time to get that permission before booking your flight late in pregnancy.

6. Ask your health care provider to suggest safe treatments for motion sickness and other common travel complaints. Also, be sure to layer your clothing, since temperature changes can shift rapidly, especially on planes.

7. Bus travel, although economical, is not usually recommended during pregnancy. Long trips can be very uncomfortable due to narrow aisles, limited bathroom space, and lack of control over rest stops.

8. Train travel, however, can be a comfortable and economical choice. Trains have more aisle space than buses or planes, rest rooms are easily accessible, and you don't have to worry about driving.

9. If you're traveling to a foreign country, carry a copy of your medical record with you, find out where medical facilities are located, and learn a bit of the medical terminology that is applicable to pregnancy in the language of the country to which you're traveling.

10. If you're traveling to a different time zone, allow a few days rest after you arrive. You may be more sensitive to jet lag while you're pregnant. Also, if you're traveling to a high altitude, relax for a couple of days to give your body a chance to adjust to the decreased oxygen.

Section Four:
What to Do the
Third Trimester

Well, you've reached the home stretch! The third trimester is a time to start tying up loose ends: complete prenatal and child care classes, make a final decision about child care, and select your baby's name. Other things you'll want to accomplish before the baby comes include selecting a pediatrician, choosing birth announcements, finishing writing baby shower thank-you notes, and attending breast-feeding classes if necessary. Don't forget also to tour the hospital labor and delivery area, postpartum rooms and nursery, pack for the hospital, and wrap up any projects at work. The waiting is almost over. . . .

CHOOSING THE RIGHT PEDIATRICIAN

Your child's doctor should be someone you respect, like, can talk to, and most of all, trust. Ask your health care provider, family, and friends for their suggestions and then interview the prospective doctor yourself in person. An informational interview is quite common. Many expectant parents want to make sure that the doctor they choose to take care of their baby is the best person for the job. This interview should be done at least four weeks before your due date, since you'll want to have your pediatrician established before you go into labor. During the interview you will get a sense of whether your philosophy of child rearing matches his or hers. Trust your instincts about whether this is the pediatrician for your family. Before the interview, ask yourself these questions:

1. Does this prospective pediatrician welcome prenatal interviews?

2. Are the office staff helpful and courteous?

3. Is the office comfortable and clean?

Use the following list of questions as a starting point in the interview process. Be sure to specifically ask about any issues that you feel strongly about.

✓ ✓ ✓ ✓ ✓ ✓ ✓ ✓ ✓ ✓ ✓ ✓ ✓ ✓ ✓
Checklist of Questions for Your Pediatrician

❍ **1.** What are your medical and pediatric qualifications?

O **2.** Which hospitals are you affiliated with?

O **3.** Are there other doctors in the group? If so, how many? What are their qualifications?

O **4.** How are phone calls handled? Whom will I speak to if you are not available?

O **5.** Do you have a call-in time for nonemergency questions?

O **6.** During an emergency or after office hours, how do I reach you?

O **7.** What are your office hours? Do you have any evening or weekend hours?

O **8.** How do you feel about working mothers? Mothers who stay at home?

O **9.** How do you feel about bottle versus breast-feeding?

O **10.** How is insurance handled? How is billing handled? When is payment expected?

O **11.** How long is the wait to schedule a routine checkup with you? Can these visits be scheduled at the time of a previous visit?

O **12.** Do you make house calls?

○ **13.** Will you come to the hospital to see my baby after it is born? If so, how soon?

THE PERFECT NAME

Choosing a name for your baby may be the hardest and most complicated part of your whole nine months. What are you going to name this soon-to-be child? Ultimately it has to please only you and your spouse, but it's nice if it also pleases both your families. In addition, you want to choose something that will be in style for the rest of your baby's life. Often choosing a name from a currently popular movie or television show may not be the best option in the long run. In order to choose the best possible name, the following category system can help organize your thoughts:

Biblical Names   Choose a name from Bible stories that mean something special to you: beautiful and sweet Rachel; gentle David and his best friend, Jonathan; and strong Joshua, who made the walls come tumbling down.

Family Names   Names of special relatives who have passed away or ones you want to honor while they are still alive make beautiful choices. Don't forget to ask about middle names. You may be surprised at what you hear! Also, think about picking a name that works well with your last name. Common rules of thumb include: 1. Choose a first name with the same number of syllables as your last name. Then choose a middle name of one less syllable than the first and last names. For example: Lyndon Baines Johnson. 2. Or try a single-syllable first name if you have a multisyllable last name. The middle name should also have two or more syllables. For example: Dwight David Eisenhower. 3. Or try multisyllable first and middle names if you have a single-syllable last name. For example: Martin Luther King.

Ethnic Names   Do you have strong ethnic roots? Honor your heritage by choosing a name popular in your family's country of origin. Try Sasha, Bruno, Maurice, Shoshanna, Olga, Jose, Tamar, or Gretchen.

Movie Star Names   Some people love Clint Eastwood or Meryl Streep. Unusual Hollywood names make excellent choices. Think of Dustin, Demi, Glenn, or Whitney. But remember, your child will have to live with this for the rest of his or her life. Be sure to choose something that you think will stand the test of time.

Royal Names   Elizabeth, George, Charles, Victoria, Nicholas, or Alexandra are all solid and regal-sounding names.

Currently Popular Names   Unisex names like Taylor, Tyler, Austin, Cody, and Jordan are popular with new parents. Other top twenty names are old standbys, like Michael, Joseph, Robert, Emily, Jennifer, and Amanda. Check with your local preschool or pediatrician's office for a list of first names. You'll get a good idea of what's hot and what's not. You also might consider giving your child a more "bread and butter" first name, but choosing a more exotic or trendy middle name that your baby can grow into.

IDEAS FOR OUR BABY'S NAME	WHOSE CHOICE	NAME ORIGIN AND MEANING
If It's a Boy		
If It's a Girl		

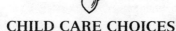

CHILD CARE CHOICES

Recently, the segment of the workforce that has increased the fastest has been moms with young babies. Since about half of all mothers with a child under one year now has a job outside the home, working mothers have become the rule rather than the exception. Choosing a caregiver can be difficult since no one can take care of your baby as well as you, but the following information about child care will help you find a high-quality caregiver and help you return to work with greater confidence and security. Before you do anything, however, you have to first decide what kind of child care you want for your baby. The type you choose will depend a lot on your lifestyle, your schedule, and your budget. Do you want your baby to stay at home with a nanny or au pair? Or do you prefer more interaction with other children at a family day care or group center? Other options available are shared family care, care by a family member, and corporate- or employee-sponsored care. Here's a look at the various options available to you:

In-Home Care

In this situation the caregiver comes to your home daily or lives in. The child receives individualized attention in familiar surroundings, but the child has no playmates. It's very convenient, but if the caregiver becomes ill, you'll need to find a backup. This form of one-on-one care tends to be the most expensive. A way to reduce the cost of in-home care is to try shared care. Shared care involves two families sharing a caregiver in one home. Parents then split the cost of an in-home caregiver. Another variant of in-home care is care by a family member. This arrangement is especially good for infants and young toddlers, since the caregiver is someone who knows and loves them. Of course, this type of care is not always an option. If you choose in-home care, you won't need to start actively looking for a caregiver until after your baby is born. Most caregivers who respond to advertisements want to start work right away.

If you're looking for an in-home caregiver, ask around for names of qualified people. Some state agencies list and certify area caregivers. Check your local phone book. Try placing an ad in the local newspaper about four weeks before you plan to return to work. You'll probably get a better response if you place the ad in several small suburban papers rather than the larger metropolitan area paper. Be general in the ad—state the age of your baby, whether you need the sitter part-time or full-time, whether you will hire someone who smokes, and the potential sitter's requirements for transportation. Screen applicants on the phone first, then meet with your top choices. During the interview, clearly state what you expect from the caregiver. Before you begin the interview, make a list of all your concerns—salary, days and hours, duties to be performed other than actual child care (e.g., laundry, light housework), benefits, and any expectations you have regarding taking the baby out of the home to the zoo, library, etc. Also ask about the caregiver's feelings about child care and discipline and knowledge of how to handle emergencies and infant/child CPR. If the person you choose is not certified in infant CPR, consider paying for them to attend a course. During the interview, watch for their response to your child and your child's response to them. If your crying baby falls asleep on the caregiver's shoulder, that's a very good sign! Ask yourself these questions: Does this person seem enthusiastic? Can I talk with her easily? Does she have a warm, caring, and patient attitude? If all your questions are answered satisfactorily, get references from parents for whom she's worked. Check *all* references carefully and trust your own instincts. Use the following checklist of questions as a guide in the interviewing process:

✓ ✓ ✓ ✓ ✓ ✓ ✓ ✓ ✓ ✓ ✓ ✓ ✓ ✓ ✓
Checklist for an In-Home Caregiver Interview

❍ **1.** What is your work history—in particular, how much experience have you had with baby care?

❍ **2.** When and why did you leave your last caregiving job?

❍ **3.** Are you interested in long-term employment?

❍ **4.** What are your fees and benefit requirements?

❍ **5.** Health history—do you have any medical problems that would make you miss work or interfere with taking care of my baby?

❍ **6.** Do you smoke, drink alcohol, or use drugs? Some parents ask their top choices to submit to a drug screening test.

❍ **7.** Do you have reliable transportation?

❍ **8.** Can you work overtime if necessary?

○ **9.** Do you anticipate any situations that might prevent you from coming to work on some days? Do you know of any backup caregivers with whom I could meet as well?

○ **10.** What things do you consider important in child rearing?

Family Child Care

This type of care takes place in the caregiver's home. In this situation your child will have other playmates, and, since the groups tend to be smaller than in larger centers, there's more chance for individual attention. Keep in mind, however, that these businesses may not be licensed by the state or monitored for proper staffing. Schedules at family centers tend to be more flexible than at larger centers, but again, if your caregiver becomes ill, you'll have to find backup care. The cost of family child care is very reasonable. If you choose family child care, you can start making plans before your baby arrives. This way, you'll have time to look at different options and, if necessary, wait for an opening.

To find quality family child care, ask friends with children, your health care provider, your church or synagogue, local community center or college, for the names of reputable facilities. Then visit that facility and ask parents of other children who attend for their opinions. Also, watch the children and babies that are there. Do they seem happy? Do the caregivers look as though they enjoy their work? Consider the following checklist of questions:

✓ ✓ ✓ ✓ ✓ ✓ ✓ ✓ ✓ ✓ ✓ ✓ ✓ ✓ ✓

Checklist for Family Child Care

○ **1.** How many children do you care for and what are their ages?

○ **2.** What are your fees?

○ **3.** How do you handle illness—your own, a family member's, or a child in your care?

○ **4.** Do you have backup help when you need it?

○ **5.** Do you carry special insurance to protect the children?

○ **6.** What are your usual hours? Do you make exceptions? Will you take care of children on weekends, holidays, or evenings if needed?

Do you take children in your car? Do you ⁓h car seats?

○ **8.** How is feeding handled? May I come during the day to nurse? Will my stored breast milk be fed to my baby? Will you feed my baby on demand or keep him or her to a schedule depending on my wishes?

○ **9.** Will you give my child any prescribed medicines?

○ **10.** Are you trained in infant CPR?

○ **11.** What are your policies on discipline? Do you ever slap, spank, or shame the children?

Make sure you spend a day observing her while she cares for the children in her home. Can she tell you about the interests and activities of the children in her care and is this someone you like and think your baby will like as well?

Center Care

In this situation children are cared for in an institutional setting. It may be sponsored by a church or synagogue, school, university, community center, social service agency, or your employer. Care tends to be less individualized

in large centers, and illness can spread quickly
from child to child. Also, the center may be
closed on holidays and probably won't accept
children with runny noses, fevers, or coughs.
Larger centers, however, usually are licensed
and monitored and provide programs suited to
your child's needs. Keep in mind that many
child care centers do not accept infants or non–
potty-trained toddlers. The cost varies based on
the program. As with family child care, if you
choose a day care center, you'll want to start
making plans before your baby arrives. Some
centers may have their infant slots filled. If your
first choice has no openings, ask to be put on a
waiting list.

✓ ✓ ✓ ✓ ✓ ✓ ✓ ✓ ✓ ✓ ✓ ✓ ✓ ✓ ✓ ✓

Checklist for Day Care Centers

◯ **1.** Is the center currently licensed or registered? Look for a license or registration on the
wall and make sure it's current. Licensure or
registration is not necessarily a guarantee of
quality.

◯ **2.** What are your regular business hours?

◯ you have a brochure or flyer showing

O **4.** Do you have a written plan for play and learning activities?

O **5.** How many babies are in the infant section? How many caregivers are in the infant section?

O **6.** On an average day, how many children come to the center?

O **7.** Can I observe before registering my baby, and am I welcome anytime my baby is there?

O **8.** How is feeding handled? Can I come to the center to nurse and/or will my breast milk be stored and fed to my baby as I wish?

O **9.** Is there a parent group and may parents come in for regular conferences?

O **10.** Does the center have a written policy on discipline?

O **11.** Is there a special area where sick children can stay until their parents arrive?

O **12.** Will the staff give prescribed medicines, and are they trained in first aid, infant CPR, and emergency procedures?

When visiting *any* child care facility, look for the following:

1. caregiver-to-child ratio

2. staff training and supervision

3. cleanliness and safety of the kitchen, sleeping, and play areas

4. age-appropriate toys and/or programs

5. sick-child policy

6. types of meals/snacks provided

7. a warm, nurturing atmosphere

8. emergency procedures

Child Care Resources
National Association of Child Care Resource and Referral Agencies
1(800)462-1600
2116 Campus Dr., S.E.
Rochester, ME 55904

National Association of Family Child Care
1(800)359-3817
725 15th St., N.W.
Suite 505
Washington, D.C. 20004

Child Care Action Campaign
1(212)239-0138
330 7th Ave., 17th floor
New York, NY 10001

Child Care Aware
1(800)424-2246

If you're going to be a stay-at-home mom, you'll also want to think about leaving your new baby with a sitter every now and then. You need the time alone and you and your partner need the time together. There are no hard and fast rules about how old an infant has to be before he or she can be left with a sitter. If you feel ready to leave your baby with a trusted sitter, there is no reason not to do it. A baby under three months of age will feel secure in the care of any responsible adult. If your baby is older than that, however, you'll want to make sure that he or she gets to meet and know the sitter before you leave. You probably should not leave your less than one year old baby with a teenager.

Whenever you leave your baby with a sitter, always make sure you provide him or her with a list of what to do and whom to call in an emergency. Always provide a phone number where you can be reached and your home address and phone number in case she needs to call 911. Use the following checklist as a guide for your sitter's reference:

✓ ✓ ✓ ✓ ✓ ✓ ✓ ✓ ✓ ✓ ✓ ✓ ✓ ✓ ✓
Baby-Sitter Checklist

I can be reached at:
Our home address and phone number:
Baby's father can be reached at:
Pediatrician's name and number:
Hospital name and number:
Fire department:
Police department:
Neighbor's name and number:
Nearest relative's name and number:
Baby's food allergies or medical problems:
Special instructions:

BIRTH ANNOUNCEMENTS:
SHARING YOUR HAPPINESS

Now is the time to begin thinking about how you want to spread the news and whom you want to tell. Your decision can be as simple as a few phone calls to special friends and family, or as elaborate as engraved announcements sent to everyone you and your families know. If you choose to send announcements through the mail, consider the following points to help you organize yourself after the baby arrives:

1. Decide whether you want to use store-bought packaged announcements that require you to fill in all vital statistics, or preprinted announcements that are created by a printer and require only that you address the envelopes. To save time, you can address your envelopes before the baby arrives. Most printers will send you your envelopes early for a small fee. If you plan on ordering at least one hundred preprinted announcements, the cost can be very comparable to packaged ones. Remember, after the baby comes you won't have much time for writing announcements, especially if you'll be writing thank-you notes for baby gifts as well.

2. Try ordering the free catalogues and birth announcement samples offered in all baby magazines. You may want to mail-order your announcements now. Or start checking out other designs at print shops, department stores, or greeting card stores.

3. All preprinted announcements can be ordered early (usually one month before your due date) and then all you have to do is call in the vital statistics right from the hospital.

4. You can either have the announcements delivered directly to your home (for a fee) or send the new dad out to pick them up.

	Call from Hospital
Name Address Phone	
Name Address Phone	
Name Address Phone	
Name Address Phone	
Name Address Phone	

	Birth Announcement	Religious-Ceremony Invitation

	Call from Hospital
Name Address Phone	
Name Address Phone	
Name Address Phone	
Name Address Phone	
Name Address Phone	

Birth Announcement	Religious-Ceremony Invitation

	Call from Hospital
Name Address Phone	
Name Address Phone	
Name Address Phone	
Name Address Phone	
Name Address Phone	

	Birth Announcement	Religious-Ceremony Invitation

	Call from Hospital
Name Address Phone	
Name Address Phone	
Name Address Phone	
Name Address Phone	
Name Address Phone	

Birth Announcement	Religious-Ceremony Invitation

	Call from Hospital
Name Address Phone	
Name Address Phone	
Name Address Phone	
Name Address Phone	
Name Address Phone	

Birth Announcement	Religious-Ceremony Invitation

5. Consider ordering thank-you notes in the same pattern as your announcements.

6. Remember to purchase stamps early so you don't have to keep running to the post office.

7. If you're having a religious ceremony after the baby arrives, such as a christening or baptism, or a bris or baby naming, decide on invitations now. Your choices remain the same between blank packaged ones or preprinted types. Consider ordering these in the same pattern as your announcements.

Note: Another option for announcements or religious-ceremony invitations is to create your own. If you're handy on a computer, you can make lovely designs and wording and then print them on special paper or cards.

Something to Celebrate: Spread the News

Use this chart to remind you whom to notify when the big day arrives. The top of the list should include whom to call from the hospital. Then expand the list to include whom to send a birth announcement to and whom to invite to any religious ceremony.

Before and after the baby arrives, many

people will be sending you gifts, from flowers to rocking horses! Since the weeks after the baby arrives can be hectic, try to keep a list of who sent what. Often the gifts come in bunches, so who a gift is from can become a blur. Sending a thank-you to Aunt Shirley for something a coworker sent can be embarrassing! Keeping a list will make life much easier and help you feel more organized when you do finally find a few minutes to relax and write a few notes. Don't forget to enclose some recent baby pictures in your thank-you notes. People love seeing just who their gift went to!

Gift	From	Date	Thank-you Note Sent

Gift	From	Date	Thank-you Note Sent

WHAT TO PACK FOR THE HOSPITAL

Although it can seem a little premature, you should begin packing now, weeks ahead of time, in order to avoid a last-minute rush. Remember, many babies are born two to three weeks before their due dates, so it's a good idea to have your bags tucked away in a closet and ready to go! As you pack, choose items that will help make your hospital stay more comfortable, personal, and familiar. Use the following three checklists of essentials to help make your hospital stay and homecoming more enjoyable and manageable.

✓ ✓ ✓ ✓ ✓ ✓ ✓ ✓ ✓ ✓ ✓ ✓ ✓ ✓ ✓
Checklist for Mom

○ **1.** A cotton nightgown or T-shirt to wear during labor. The hospital will undoubtedly provide you with a hospital gown, but you may feel more comfortable in your own clothes.

○ **2.** Two nightgowns (with button fronts for nursing or bring nursing pajamas). Some women prefer to wear the hospital gown after labor to avoid staining their new nighties.

○ **3.** A warm bed jacket or robe for walking the hospital halls

○ **4.** Nonskid slippers

○ **5.** 2 bras (nursing bras for nursing moms)

○ **6.** 4 pairs of maternity panties

○ **7.** Thick socks, since cold feet are common during labor

○ **8.** Toiletries: comb and brush; toothbrush; toothpaste; soap; shampoo; lip balm; lotion; hair dryer; deodorant; and breath-freshening spray (for during labor to keep your mouth fresh and moist)

○ **9.** Eyeglasses or contact lenses and cases. You can wear glasses during labor, but you'll need to remove contact lenses.

○ **10.** Hair band, ponytail holder, or barrettes to tie hair back during labor

○ **11.** Sanitary napkins designed for extra heavy flow (if the hospital does not provide them)

○ **12.** An extra bed pillow (with nonwhite pillowcase) for your comfort during labor

O **13.** Favorite object or photo to focus on during labor—try a relaxing nature picture to hang on the wall or your baby's first toy to hold

O **14.** Sugar-free lollipops or fruit drops to keep your mouth moist during labor

O **15.** A box of dried fruit for postpartum constipation

O **16.** Light reading for early labor

O **17.** Postlabor feel-good perks: your favorite lipstick or other makeup, revitalizing shower gel, perfume, or scented powder

O **18.** Going-home outfit—about the size you wore in your fifth month

O **19.** Small, inexpensive gifts for postpartum nurses. Or order a gift basket for all the nurses to share. You may want to get something special for your labor and delivery nurse if she gave you one-on-one care and was with you for the majority of your labor and birth. This can be purchased later and sent to her at the hospital when you know she'll be on duty.

O **20.** Gift for your firstborn from the baby

✓ ✓ ✓ ✓ ✓ ✓ ✓ ✓ ✓ ✓ ✓ ✓ ✓ ✓ ✓ ✓

Checklist for Baby

○ **1.** Receiving blanket

○ **2.** Diapers (if the hospital doesn't provide them)

○ **3.** A car seat—you can't drive your baby home without one

○ **4.** Going-home outfit: undershirt, newborn sleeper, hat/cap, bunting or jacket (depending on the season), socks

○ **5.** Heavier blanket (depending on the season)

✓ ✓ ✓ ✓ ✓ ✓ ✓ ✓ ✓ ✓ ✓ ✓ ✓ ✓ ✓ ✓

Checklist for Dad

○ **1.** Insurance and hospital preregistration information

○ **2.** Watch or clock with a second hand to time contractions

○ **3.** Change of clothes. If Dad is allowed to room in on a cot or pullout couch after the baby comes, he should bring enough clothes, underwear, etc., for several days.

O **4.** Razor and all toiletries

O **5.** Support items during labor: lotion or powders for massage, tennis balls in a sock or a rolling pin for lower back massage, soothing music (tapes or CDs) with a portable tape or CD player, this book and a pen to jot down thoughts during labor or make a to-do list (use the notes section at the end), childbirth preparation manual, colored washcloth for your forehead

O **6.** Personal phone book and a must-call list (use the list from this book). Bring long distance calling card and plenty of pocket change. Also give him your work phone number so he can call to tell them you're in labor.

O **7.** Phone number of the stationery store to call in vital statistics for preselected birth announcements

O **8.** Camera and film, video recorder and tapes, and/or blank audiotape and cassette recorder for recording the birth and for after the happy event. Be sure to check the batteries before you pack and what type of equipment the hospital allows.

O **9.** Plenty of nonperishable snacks. Don't bring anything with a very strong aroma,

which could make you hungry or nauseated
during labor.

○ **10.** A bottle of champagne or other celebra-
tory food/drink! Even a nursing mother can
have one small glass of champagne to celebrate
the birth of her baby. Other foods like sweets,
pizza, or any favorite dish can be served!!

BUILDING YOUR SUPPORT NETWORK

It's important to have help after your baby arrives. New mothers should take full advantage
of their maternity leaves. Don't try to do too
many things, other than taking care of your
newborn, too soon. Maternity leave is a time to
concentrate on your baby and leave everything
else to other people. Remember, your baby will
be a newborn only for a short time—these are
precious moments that should not be wasted.
Bringing in help is a way to maintain calm in
your household. Sometimes it will be your
mother or mother-in-law or both. Other relatives, friends, or your husband can serve as
your postpartum helper. Another choice is to
hire a baby nurse or doulah for your first few
weeks home. A doulah is a helper who special-
izes in taking care of the new mother by reliev-

ing her of household chores that take time away from caring for new baby. Regardless of whom you choose to help you after the baby arrives, make sure he or she knows exactly what his or her role is regarding household chores and baby care. Do you want him or her to do all the middle-of-the-night feedings? Or are you planning to nurse and would prefer he or she help you out by cooking and cleaning? Make sure roles are clearly defined to avoid hassles during the stressful time when you're adjusting to new parenthood.

If friends and relatives call to ask how they can help in your final few weeks of pregnancy, have them choose a task from the following checklist:

✓ ✓ ✓ ✓ ✓ ✓ ✓ ✓ ✓ ✓ ✓ ✓ ✓ ✓ ✓ ✓ ✓
Help-in-the-Final-Weeks Checklist

○ **1.** Help with pre-baby housecleaning. You may also want to consider hiring a service to clean before your baby arrives home.

○ **2.** Prepare and freeze casseroles and stews or bring meals after the baby arrives. Another idea for help with meals is to check out local restaurants that deliver and keep their phone numbers and menus handy.

○ **3.** Help address birth announcements.

○ **4.** Be a backup person to take you to the hospital.

○ **5.** Telephone other friends or family with the good news.

○ **6.** Care for pets and plants while you're in the hospital.

○ **7.** Take in mail and newspapers while you're in the hospital.

○ **8.** Care for older children during and after your hospital stay.

○ **9.** Promise to baby-sit after you come home from the hospital.

○ **10.** Run last-minute errands—to the drugstore for sanitary pads (an essential after delivery), lip balm and breath-freshening spray (for use during labor to moisten your mouth), or to the grocery store for dried fruit (to eat in the hospital after delivery to help relieve the inevitable constipation).

In building your support network, don't be surprised to find that your relationships with your friends change as you get closer to delivery. Friends without children may feel ambivalent or left out as you begin to make new

friends with other pregnant women and mothers, and single friends often worry that there
will be no time left for friendship after your
baby arrives. Although most friends are very
interested in the upcoming new addition to
your family, try to keep in mind that your
friends have as much going on in their lives
now as they did before you had your baby! Always ask how things are going and continue to
make time for them—both with and without
your baby. While some friends may grow dis-
tant for a while, if you make an extra effort to
keep in touch, they will be back as they adjust to
your new life.

TYING UP LOOSE ENDS
AND PLANNING AHEAD

In addition to building your support network,
here are some details you can attend to in the
weeks before your baby is due that will make
your trip to the hospital, your short stay, and
your return home much easier. Don't forget to
pay attention to details and get "all your ducks
in a row" both at home and at work *before* the
big day!

✓ ✓ ✓ ✓ ✓ ✓ ✓ ✓ ✓ ✓ ✓ ✓ ✓ ✓ ✓ ✓
The Countdown Checklist

○ **1.** Confirm your due date with your pediatrician and make certain your health care provider knows the name and number of your pediatrician.

○ **2.** Plan and time your route to the hospital. Find the quickest way to the hospital and know how long the trip will take. Figure in rush hour traffic or bad weather conditions. You may even want to take practice runs at various times of the day and in varied weather conditions. Plan an alternate route in case of delay.

○ **3.** Take a tour of the labor and delivery area of your hospital. Ask about the hospital's visiting hours, waiting area for family, which entrance to use, how to get in if you arrive in labor late at night, which elevator to use, policy on using the emergency room during labor, and specifically what supplies the hospital will provide you and the baby (e.g., sanitary napkins or diapers).

○ **4.** Ask about preregistration. Bring insurance information to the hospital tour and try to preregister at this time.

○ **5.** Establish a backup person to take you to the hospital or have the phone number of a twenty-four-hour taxi service handy.

○ **6.** Make child care arrangements for older children. Try to rely on a nearby friend or relative, since you could go into labor late at night.

○ **7.** Rent a baby beeper to notify your partner when you're in labor. Most businesses that sell or rent beepers have special baby beeper programs that provide short-term beeper use for a minimal price.

○ **8.** Install the car seat. Make sure you and your partner practice using the infant car seat before you try to work it with your newborn. A cushion insert that supports a newborn's fragile head and neck can make the ride home more comfortable.

○ **9.** Purchase two weeks worth of staples for the kitchen. Clean out a kitchen shelf for bottles and other baby-feeding paraphernalia.

○ **10.** Purchase and wrap small gifts for your older children to get from the baby on your return from the hospital.

○ **11.** Finish all baby shower thank-you notes.

A WORD ABOUT THE FAMILY PET

Prepare your pet for the baby's homecoming by giving him something that the new baby has worn. Many veterinarians recommend using the neonatal hat, which will have the baby's scent on it. Let your pet adjust to the smell and then introduce the baby to him. He may seem curious or indifferent. Animals do not like change in their routines. If you normally walk him in the mornings or feed him at a certain time, continue to do so. This will help make his adjustment easier and reduce the likelihood of jealousy. Watch for any signs of aggression, however, and be sure to let the animal know that the baby is a part of the family. Reprimand any aggressive behaviors immediately. No matter how docile or friendly your pet may be, never leave your baby unattended in a room with any animal.

LIST OF IMPORTANT NUMBERS
TO KEEP HANDY

Health Care Provider:
  Office:
  Answering Service:

Hospital:
  Main Number:
  Labor and Delivery:
Taxi Service:
Local Pharmacy:
Insurance Company:
  Phone No.:
  Group #:
  ID #:
  My Social Security Number:
  Spouse's Social Security Number:
Pediatrician:
  Office:
  Answering Service:
Day Care:
Baby-Sitters:
  1.
  2.
  3.
Fire:
911
Poison Control:

Section Five:
Postpartum—The First
Six Weeks

IT'S A . . . BABY

All your planning has paid off! You have a beautiful new addition to your family and your home is all set to welcome him or her. Following is postpartum information on everything from what to ask before you leave the hospital to what to ask at your baby's six-month checkup, all guaranteed to help make this wonderful time worry-free. Just ahead, also, is a section for you to jot down special memories and information about the day your baby was born.

MEMORABLE KEEPSAKES OF YOUR
BABY'S BIRTH DAY

Happy Birthday, _____!

Birth date:

Time:

Location:

Delivered by:

Nurse:

Special support person:

Describe labor and delivery:

    Labor began at:

    We went to the hospital at:

    The weather was:

    Length of labor:

    Music I listened to:

    My focal point was:

    When my baby was born I felt:

Apgar scores: at 1 minute: at 5 minutes:

Birth weight: lbs.   oz.

Length:

Head circumference:

Hair color:

Eye color:

Any birthmarks:

Blood type/Rh:

GET THE FACTS BEFORE YOU LEAVE THE HOSPITAL

You'll always remember that first trip home from the hospital with your new baby. It's a memory universally shared by new parents. To make the trip home less stressful and more enjoyable, make sure you have as much information as you can get before you leave the hospital. Plan to ask the postpartum nurses the following questions and request that they give you all information in writing. You'll have a lot on your mind and probably won't remember everything they tell you.

✓ ✓ ✓ ✓ ✓ ✓ ✓ ✓ ✓ ✓ ✓ ✓ ✓ ✓ ✓
Checklist of Questions to Ask Before You Leave the Hospital

❍ **1.** How do I care for my stitches?

❍ **2.** How do I handle postpartum concerns like pain and constipation?

❍ **3.** What type of breast-feeding tips can you provide me? If a lactation nurse is available, try to meet with her at least once before you leave and get her phone number for later use. Some hospitals have a twenty-four-hour lactation consultant hotline.

○ **4.** What type of newborn care tips can you give me? Newborn care tips include how to care for the umbilical cord stump and/or circumcision, and how to change a diaper and give a sponge bath. Practice newborn care in the hospital.

○ **5.** What unusual symptoms, for me or my baby, should I report to my health care provider or the baby's pediatrician? Most illnesses your baby will get are minor and will require no special medical treatment. But don't hesitate to call the doctor if your intuition tells you to or in case of any of the following:

✓ ✓ ✓ ✓ ✓ ✓ ✓ ✓ ✓ ✓ ✓ ✓ ✓ ✓ ✓
Checklist for When to Call the Pediatrician

○ **1.** Temperature of 101 degrees F under three months old

○ **2.** Temperature over 102 degrees F over three months

○ **3.** Lethargic, difficult to rouse

○ **4.** Difficulty breathing

○ **5.** Refusal to drink liquids

○ **6.** Excessive diarrhea or vomiting

○ **7.** Signs of dehydration: little urination, no tears, dry mouth, doughy skin

○ **8.** Persistent and inexplicable crying

○ **9.** Febrile seizure

CARING FOR YOUR NEWBORN

Now that you're home from the hospital, you're on! There seems to be a million new tasks for you to do all at once, and as a new mom you're probably concerned about doing everything exactly right. Relax! Although the responsibility may seem overwhelming at first, with time, *practice,* and experience you'll learn what makes your baby happy and keeps him or her comfortable. Taking care of your new baby is the hardest job you'll ever love! Following are some helpful tips for the daily tasks involved in caring for your little one.

Diaper Changing

1. Change diapers often to reduce the exposure of baby's tender skin to harmful substances in urine and stool. If baby develops a diaper rash, apply an ointment containing zinc oxide. If the rash doesn't heal within two or three days, call the pediatrician.

2. Have all your diapering supplies within reach. Never leave your baby unattended on a changing surface even for an instant, since he or she could roll off.

3. Wet diapers: Clean baby with an alcohol-free premoistened wipe, a damp cotton ball or soft cloth, or baby oil. Pat dry and apply either a moisture-barrier ointment like A and D or petroleum jelly or talc-free baby powder or pure cornstarch. Always pour the powder into your hand before applying to baby to prevent baby from inhaling the powder particles. If you're using disposable diapers with adhesive tabs, be sure to wipe your hand thoroughly before trying to close the tabs. Any oily substance will prevent the tabs from sticking.

4. Dirty diapers: Clean baby with alcohol-free premoistened wipes or a soapy washcloth. Always clean a girl from front to back (clean to dirty) and leave an uncircumcised boy's fore-skin alone. Apply ointments or powders as with wet diapers.

5. Keep the umbilical cord area as clean and dry as you can. Drip alcohol from a cotton ball or cotton swab into the wet, unhealed area to promote drying and healing. The cord stump usually drops off within ten days to two weeks after birth but may not fall off for a month. If the area oozes or the skin becomes reddened, call your pediatrician. Fold the diaper down so it doesn't rub on the healing area, or if you're using disposable diapers, choose newborn ones that have a bellybutton cutout.

Burping

1. Hold baby upright against your shoulder. This will allow the air in baby's stomach to rise above the milk and escape. Some baby's prefer to be burped lying on their stomachs on your lap.

2. Rub or pat him or her gently on the back. Sometimes rubbing in an upward motion on the back encourages the air to come up and out.

3. Don't shake your baby around while burping, as this will cause the air and milk to mix together and both will come out.

4. Don't try to burp your baby if he or she is still sucking or sleeping. When your baby does need to burp, he or she will let you know.

Sponge Bathing

1. Don't bathe your newborn more than every other day, and for the first week use water only—no soap.

2. Clean baby's face every day and diaper area at every changing.

3. Bathe your baby before he or she eats to avoid spit-up and bowel movements during the bath.

4. Keep the room where you bathe baby at about 75 degrees F.

5. Gather all supplies ahead of time. Use the following checklist: mild, unscented soap; washcloth; cotton balls; receiving blanket; one large towel; alcohol (for cleaning the cord stump); ointment; clean diaper; clean clothes or pajamas.

6. Have two bowls of water nearby—one for a soapy washcloth and one for rinse water. You don't need a sink area for a sponge bath.

7. Keep the baby dressed while you clean his or her hair and scalp, eyes (clean from inside out with a cotton ball), ears, nose, face, and neck. Never use a cotton swab in ears or nose. Pat dry completely, especially the back and creases of the neck.

8. Undress the baby and wrap him or her in the receiving blanket, making sure to keep his or her head covered. Thoroughly wash the entire body, paying special attention to the creases. Expose only the part of the body being washed to avoid chilling baby.

9. Clean the cord stump with alcohol and a cotton ball. This should also be done at all diaper changes until it falls off. You may give your baby a tub bath after the cord has healed.

10. Always clean a girl's genitals from front to back (clean to dirty); when cleaning a boy's uncircumcised penis, never pull back on the foreskin unless you get the okay from your pediatri-

cian; your pediatrician will also tell you how to
care for a circumcised penis.

Dressing

1. Always use clothes that open to the front to
avoid having to turn baby over.

2. A receiving blanket laid over your baby's
bare skin will help keep him or her feeling comfortable as you dress other areas.

3. If you're using an undershirt or onesie,
bunch it up in both hands to expand the neck
opening before putting it over baby's head.

4. Help sleeves go on more easily by reaching
into each sleeve from the end the hand comes
out of and gently pulling baby's arm through.

5. Use a bib on baby before feedings to mini-
mize clothing changes.

Nail Cutting

1. Use baby scissors with rounded ends or
baby nail clippers. Never try to cut a newborn's
nails with regular scissors or nail clippers.

2. Clip the nail short to keep baby from scratching him- or herself.

3. Try to cut baby's nails when he or she is sleeping to prevent accidental cuts from squirming.

4. Hold baby's hand so that his or her fingers and yours point in the same direction.

5. Baby's fingernails will grow much faster than his or her toenails. You'll probably need to cut his or her fingernails at least once a week, while the toenails may need to be cut only once a month.

Taking a Temperature

1. Shake thermometer until the mercury line is below 96 degrees F (for *mercury* rectal or oral thermometers only).

2. Put the bulb end of *any kind* of thermometer under baby's armpit with baby's arm held snugly against his/her body. This is called an axillary temperature.

3. Be sure the thermometer is between skin and skin, not clothing.

4. Hold the thermometer in place for three to seven minutes before removing.

5. To read the thermometer, hold it in both hands, one at each end, and slowly rotate it until the mercury can be seen between the numbers and lines. Read the temperature where the mercury ends. Read the number that is to the left of the end of the mercury line, then add two points for each little line between the number and the end of the mercury line.

6. Normal axillary temperature is 97.6 degrees F. Fever is when the axillary temperature reads 99 degrees F and above. A high fever is when the axillary temperature is 104 degrees F.

An Update on Preventing SIDS

One of the most frightening possibilities for new parents is sudden infant death syndrome (SIDS), where an otherwise healthy baby dies for no apparent reason. SIDS occurs most frequently in infants ages two to four months. Though no one knows the causes of SIDS, removing the risk factors associated with it has helped decrease the number of SIDS deaths. The following set of guidelines for preventing

SIDS is recommended by the American Academy of Pediatrics:

1. Place baby on his or her side or back to sleep.

2. If baby must sleep on his or her stomach, do the following: unswaddle the baby from the receiving blanket and use a firm mattress without a pillow or other soft bedding.

3. Avoid overheating baby's room and have baby wear as many layers of clothing as you would be comfortable in plus one extra layer, such as a receiving blanket (wrapped loosely around baby).

4. Never smoke around baby (before or after birth). Do not permit anyone else to smoke around baby either.

Care Essentials for Your Newborn

In addition to the new tasks you'll be facing, it also seems like you suddenly need an enormous amount of toiletries and sundries just to get through a day! For as small as they are, babies certainly do take up a lot of space in your home. The following newborn care checklist can serve as a handy reminder of the numerous essentials required to keep your baby clean and healthy. Pre-purchasing many of these fundamentals can help keep you from being caught short when you get your newborn home. Remember to have extras for your diaper bag.

✓ ✓ ✓ ✓ ✓ ✓ ✓ ✓ ✓ ✓ ✓ ✓ ✓ ✓ ✓

Newborn Care Checklist

○ **1.** Petroleum jelly or A and D ointment

○ **2.** Zinc oxide ointment

○ **3.** Alcohol-free premoistened wipes

○ **4.** Baby oil

○ **5.** Baby lotion

○ **6.** Alcohol for care of the cord stump

○ **7.** Cotton balls

○ **8.** Cotton swabs (only for cleaning the cord area)

○ **9.** Talc-free baby powder or pure cornstarch

○ **10.** Mild liquid or bar soap

○ **11.** Baby brush and comb (with rounded ends)

○ **12.** Baby nail scissors (with rounded tips) or baby nail clippers

○ **13.** Baby shampoo

○ **14.** Digital or mercury thermometer

○ **15.** Bulb syringe for cleaning mucus from baby's nose and mouth

○ **16.** Medicine dropper for giving any medicines

○ **17.** Baby sun screen

CALMING A FUSSY BABY

Coping with crying is one of the biggest challenges a new parent must face. It's so frustrating when a baby cries and you don't know why. A crying baby can make you feel helpless, inadequate, or even angry. Try this checklist of soothers. Go down the list and see what works for your baby:

○ **1.** Offer breast or bottle. Hunger is the most common cause of crankiness.

○ **2.** Check baby's diaper. Change a dirty diaper and check for diaper rash. Some babies cry when they are having a bowel movement.

○ **3.** If the problem is diaper rash, remove the diaper and let baby go undressed for a short while. This will lessen any chafing and air can actually help the healing process.

○ **4.** Check to see if baby is too hot or too cold. He or she should be dressed in the same weight clothes as you are (with one additional layer such as a receiving blanket) to be comfortable.

○ **5.** Hold baby's ear close to your heart. The sound of your heartbeat and breathing is familiar and soothing. Also try this with your baby undressed next to your bare skin. Skin-to-skin contact has a very calming effect.

○ **6.** Lay baby on his or her back and gently "bicycle" his or her legs. This can help relieve gas pains.

○ **7.** Lay baby tummy-down across your knees and move your knees up and down.

○ **8.** Try a pacifier. Some babies need the comfort of sucking.

○ **9.** Wear your baby in a front carrier. The movement seems to calm many babies.

○ **10.** Wrap baby in a receiving blanket. Some babies feel more snug and secure when swaddled.

○ **11.** Give baby a warm bath, gently massaging his or her tummy. This will re-create the sensation of being in the womb.

○ **12.** Place baby tummy-down on a folded towel that's been warmed in the dryer. Massage his or her back to help an upset tummy.

○ **13.** Play soothing music from a tape player or music box.

○ **14.** Use a rocking chair or glider. Babies like the rhythmic motion.

○ **15.** Place baby tummy-down on a folded towel or blanket on top of the running washer or dryer. Keep a good hold on him or her at all times. The motion and noise will soothe your baby.

○ **16.** Try "white noise" from a vacuum cleaner, running water, or the static between radio stations. No one knows why, but these monotonous sounds calm some fussy babies.

○ **17.** Place baby near a window so he or she can look out and hopefully be distracted.

○ **18.** Place baby in a mechanical infant swing. During the busy dinner hour, this can be a life saver!

○ **19.** Take baby for a stroller or carriage ride outdoors. The motion, change of scenery, and fresh air can soothe an irritable baby.

○ **20.** Strap baby securely into the car seat and take a lulling drive. This is one of the most surefire options.

○ **21.** If you're breast-feeding, think about what you've been eating. Certain foods in your diet may be causing gas in your baby. Garlic, onions, broccoli, and cabbage are common culprits.

○ **22.** If you're bottle feeding, consider switching formulas. Always check with your pediatrician before changing types of formula. Also, check the temperature of the bottle. Some babies prefer warm versus cool bottles, or vice versa.

○ **23.** Some babies need to be left alone in a safe, quiet room (in their crib, of course) when they are overstimulated. Ask your pediatrician how to and if you should go about letting the baby "cry it out."

VISITING THE PEDIATRICIAN

Well-baby visits give you and your pediatrician the opportunity to ask questions and get information regarding your baby's growth and development, eating and sleeping patterns, and general health. Your doctor will ask questions relating to age-appropriate milestones to check for proper development and perform a complete physical exam. Well-baby visits are also an important time for your baby to receive the required immunizations to keep him or her healthy. Although the timing of these visits is fairly standard, each pediatrician's schedule may vary slightly. Always check with your doctor to make sure your baby is seen at the right time. The following two charts will help you keep track of these regular physical exams and the immunizations your baby needs.

Keep a record of your baby's immunizations on the following chart. You may need such a record when your child enters school, and it can serve as a convenient reference in later years. The following schedule of immunizations is recommended by the American Academy of Pediatrics for healthy infants and children. Your child should be fully immunized by age of two. In special circumstances, your pediatrician may suggest a different schedule for your child. If you have any questions or concerns, please contact your pediatrician.

YOUR SIX-WEEK
POSTPARTUM CHECKUP

At your six-week postpartum checkup your health care provider will want to make sure that you are making a healthy recovery. He or she will check your uterus to make sure it is returning to normal size, probably do a pap test, ask you how you're feeling emotionally to check for postpartum blues or depression, and discuss various birth control or family planning options with you if you don't want to get pregnant again right away. It is a myth that you can't conceive right after having a baby. If you are bottle feeding, your menstruation will probably return by your six-week checkup. If you are nursing, menstruation will not return until you stop. Some women do not get a period for a year or more.

✓ ✓ ✓ ✓ ✓ ✓ ✓ ✓ ✓ ✓ ✓ ✓ ✓ ✓ ✓ ✓

Checklist of Questions to Ask at Your Six-Week Postpartum Checkup

○ **1.** When can I have intercourse with my partner again? You should not have intercourse until after your six-week checkup.

○ **2.** Which option for birth control or family planning do you recommend for me? If the birth control method you choose requires a prescription, don't forget to ask for it before you leave the office. Refer to the following chart before your appointment so that you have your choices in mind.

○ **3.** What can I do about sore breasts or nipples as a result of breast-feeding?

○ **4.** Should I still take my prenatal vitamin or any other supplement?

○ **5.** Is my recovery normal?

○ **6.** When can I start exercising? Are there any limitations on my exercise?

WELL-BABY CHECKUP CHART

Age	Date	Weight	
2-week checkup			
2-month checkup			
4-month checkup			
6-month checkup			

	Length	Head Circumference	Lab Results

WELL-BABY CHECKUP CHART

Age	Date	Weight	
9-month checkup			
12-month checkup			
15-month checkup			
18-month checkup			
24-month checkup			

	Length	Head Circumference	Lab Results

IMMUNIZATIONS RECORD

Immunization	Recommended Ages	
DTP (Diphtheria, tetanus, and pertussis)	2 months 4 months 6 months 15 to 18 months 4 to 6 years	
Oral Polio	2 months 4 months 6 to 18 months 4 to 6 years	
MMR (measles, mumps, rubella	12 to 15 months 4 to 6 years (in certain areas) 11 to 12 years	

Actual Date Given	Physician or Health Care Facility Providing Care

IMMUNIZATIONS RECORD

Immunization	Recommended Ages
Hepatitis B (HBV)	Birth 1 to 2 months 6 to 18 months
Varicella (Chicken Pox—Optional)	12 months or older
HIB (Hemophilus B influenza)	2 months 4 months 6 months 12 to 15 months
Tetanus-Diphtheria (Td)	14 to 16 years
Other	

	Actual Date Given	Physician or Health Care Facility Providing Care

○ **7.** What can I do about postpartum blues?

○ **8.** How much weight have I lost and what do you recommend as a healthy weight for me?

○ **9.** When do I need to make a return visit?

○ **10.** When will my normal energy levels return?

BIRTH CONTROL CHOICES AND THE NEW MOTHER

One of the first questions a new mother may want to ask her health care provider is what to do about contraception. Most experts believe that a woman can become pregnant as early as four weeks after giving birth if she is not nursing. If you don't want another child immediately, now is the time to decide what kind of family planning to use. There is no correct method, but there are a number of factors to consider. The method you choose must be safe, effective, and, if you want more children, reversible. The choice that's best for you will depend on your health, physical condition, and personal preference.

EXERCISING WITH YOUR NEW BABY

Many new mothers find that the best way to shed those pregnancy pounds is to walk with their babies. It's easy, convenient, stimulating for your baby, and you won't have to worry about a baby-sitter or child care! Several companies make specially designed exercise strollers for this purpose. You don't need a fancy, expensive stroller, however, to enjoy walking with your baby. Any sturdy stroller that has handles at a comfortable height for you and a place to store a few essential items will do just fine. The following tips and information will help if you decide to walk off those pounds with your new baby in tow.

✓ ✓ ✓ ✓ ✓ ✓ ✓ ✓ ✓ ✓ ✓ ✓ ✓ ✓ ✓ ✓
Postpartum Walking Checklist

○ **1.** Be sure to get a good pair of walking shoes. Keep in mind that your feet may have changed sizes since being pregnant.

○ **2.** If you've walked previously, maintain your regular speed and distance, as walking with a stroller burns more calories.

BIRTH CONTROL CHOICES

Method	Effectiveness	
Birth Control Pill	94–99.9%	
Spermicide (alone)	79–97%	
Condom (alone)	88–98%	
Diaphragm (with spermicide)	82–94%	
Contraceptive Sponge	72–94%	

Advantages	Disadvantages
1. Allows for sexual spontaneity 2. Helps protect against ovarian and endometrial cancer 3. Reduces menstrual irregularities and PID (pelvic inflammatory disease) risk	1. Must be taken daily 2. No sexually transmitted disease (STD) protection 3. Increases risk of blood clots, heart attack, stroke, especially in smokers over thirty-five
1. Inexpensive 2. Helps protect against some STDs	1. Reduces sexual spontaneity 2. Messy, reapplication required for repeated intercourse 3. May increase risk of urinary tract infections
1. Inexpensive 2. Helps protect against STDs	1. Reduces sexual spontaneity 2. May reduce sensation 3. Breakage rate: 1 out of 160
1. Helps protect against STDs 2. Lowers PID risk 3. Can insert up to 6 hours before intercourse	1. Reduces sexual spontaneity 2. Increases risk of urinary tract and bladder infections
1. Inexpensive 2. 24-hour protection	1. One time use only 2. Can cause dryness 3. **Less effective in women with children**

Method	Effectiveness	
Contraceptive Implant System	98.8%	
Intrauterine Device (IUD)	97–99.9%	
Tubal Ligation (tied tubes)	99.6–99.8%	
Vasectomy	99.85–99.9%	
Natural Family Planning (periodic abstinence)	80–99%	

Advantages	Disadvantages
1. Allows sexual spontaneity 2. Five-year protection 3. Completely reversible	1. Menstrual irregularities 2. No STD protection
1. Allows sexual spontaneity 2. Effective for one to six years, depending on type	1. Menstrual problems 2. Increases PID risk with multiple partners 3. May be expelled or perforate uterus 4. No STD protection
1. Allows sexual spontaneity 2. Permanent outpatient surgical procedure	1. Expensive 2. Usually irreversible 3. Surgical risk 4. No STD protection
1. Allows sexual spontaneity 2. Minor surgery (as compared to tubal ligation)	1. Expensive 2. Usually irreversible 3. Surgical risk 4. No STD protection
1. Free 2. No artificial means of pregnancy prevention	1. Careful monitoring of a woman's temperature and cervical mucous required 2. Reduces sexual spontaneity 3. No STD protection

○ **3.** Bring along essential supplies such as bottles of juice, breast milk, or formula; diapers and wipes; and water for yourself. Nursing moms may want to feed their babies just before they walk to allow lactic acid (which builds up during exercise) to leave their systems before the next feeding. Lactic acid sometimes makes nursing babies fussy.

○ **4.** Don't let your baby distract you from walking safely—pay attention to your environment. Watch especially for hazards to your baby like flying road debris, extreme noise, or smoke and dust. Never walk with headphones.

○ **5.** If you let go of the stroller, always lock the rear brake.

○ **6.** Dress your baby appropriately. Remember he or she won't be exercising, so may need to be dressed more warmly than you are.

○ **7.** Choose a walking plan that's right for you. You can adhere to a strict walking regimen with calculated speeds and distances, or you can just choose any destination and briskly walk there and back (enjoying the scenery along the way!).

TRAVELING WITH YOUR BABY

Traveling with your baby can seem like a daunting experience. Whether it's a day trip to the zoo or a cross-country flight, packing and carrying your baby's things (all the extra stuff you now have to lug with you) will seem like the most challenging part! The following checklist of the most useful products designed to make traveling with baby easier should help.

✓ ✓ ✓ ✓ ✓ ✓ ✓ ✓ ✓ ✓ ✓ ✓ ✓ ✓ ✓ ✓
Traveling with Baby Checklist

○ **1.** Your well-stocked diaper bag. The *most* essential item!

○ **2.** An infant carrier or backpack (for an older baby). This allows your hands to be free.

○ **3.** Powdered baby formula that can be mixed with tap water at the feeding time and therefore doesn't need refrigeration or warming. Keep several bottles filled with warm or cool tap water for use throughout the day.

○ **4.** A small cooler for snacks, bottles, juice, and pumped breast milk.

○ **5.** A first aid kit, including bandages, a thermometer, baby acetaminophen, any prescription medication for baby, antibacterial ointment, your pediatrician's name and phone number.

○ **6.** A lightweight umbrella stroller for running through airports, or city walking tours. Remember, don't use a sling-back type of umbrella stroller until your baby can be propped comfortably.

○ **7.** A childproofing kit containing outlet covers, night-light, safety latches for windows, electrical cord shorteners, and toilet locks for overnight stays.

○ **8.** A portable crib or play yard. Many hotels do not provide cribs to families. Check ahead of time to see if you need to bring this item with you.

○ **9.** A car seat duffel bag especially for carrying the car seat through busy airports.

PLAYING WITH YOUR BABY

Although it may seem like all your baby does in the first few months is eat, sleep, and cry, babies are learning and absorbing all the time. Here are some simple games you can play together to begin stimulating your baby mentally and physically.

Games Babies Love to Play

1. Peek-a-boo (Cover your face with your hands and say "Where's Mommy," then uncover your face and say, "Peek-a-boo, I see you!")

2. Sooo big (Say, "How big is baby? Sooo big!" Then spread your arm wide and repeat.)

3. Clap hands or **hurray** or pat-a-cake (Pat-a-cake, pat-a-cake, baker's man/Bake me a cake as fast as you can/You pat it, you roll it, you mark it with a B/And you put it in the oven for baby and me!)

4. Open/shut (Open and close your fingers, repeating open, shut.)

5. Itsy-bitsy spider (Move fingers upward in a spider motion, make rain come down with your fingers, make the sun come up with your arms, and make the spider crawl up again while singing: "The itsy-bitsy spider crawled up the garden spout/Down came the rain and washed the spider out/Out came the sun and dried up all the rain/And the itsy-bitsy spider crawled up the spout again.")

6. Bicycle song ("I bicycle here, I bicycle there, I bicycle bicycle everywhere"—bicycle baby's legs—"with a kick and a boom, a kick and a boom, a kick and a boom and hurray!" Gently kick and rock baby's legs.)

7. Animal sounds (Say, "How does a doggie go? Woof-woof. How does a cow go? Moo-moo.")

8. Use rattles and squeaky toys to stimulate baby's senses

9. Sing lullabies to your baby

10. Read to your baby

Young Babies' Favorite Things to Look At

1. Your face (always the most favorite)

2. Color contrasts (mainly black and white)

3. Black dots on a white background

4. Broad stripes

5. Bull's-eyes

6. Checkerboards

7. Black and white photos (especially of Mom's and Dad's faces)

8. Ceiling fans or ceiling beams

9. Fires in fireplaces

10. Silhouettes

Section Six:
Pregnancy Calendar

HOW TO USE
THE PREGNANCY CALENDAR

The following pregnancy calendar is designed to help you keep track of all your important appointments and to simplify your overwhelming to-do list during the forty weeks of pregnancy. Fill in the name of the appropriate month and the corresponding dates according to your individual pregnancy. There is also space for you to track your monthly weight gain (to make sure it's not too much or too little) and a place to jot down questions for your health care provider as you think of them. Each month also has reminders of important checklist items to accomplish during that month. It should help to keep you on track, organized, and relaxed until the big day! Remember to bring this book and calendar to all your health care provider appointments and even on shopping trips for maternity clothes, layette items, and baby furnishings.

In conclusion, I wish you an easy labor and

a healthy baby, and I promise you that you will survive both childbirth and child rearing. Remember, every child is different and so is every parent. In the end, you'll succeed if you use love, care, and good sense, and if you listen to your heart.

From my family to yours, best wishes for a happy, healthy pregnancy and a joyous life with your new baby!

The Pregnancy Calendar
MONTH: _____

FIRST MONTH OF PREGNANCY

SUNDAY	MONDAY	TUESDAY	WEDNESDAY	THURSDAY	FRIDAY	SATURDAY
START EATING HEALTHY FOODS NOW ☐	☐	☐	QUIT SMOKING NOW ☐	☐	☐	☐
☐	☐	☐	☐	☐	☐	☐
CONCEPTION PROBABLY OCCURRED THIS WEEK ☐	☐	☐	☐	☐	☐	☐
☐	☐	☐	☐	☐	☐	☐
KEEP IMPORTANT PHONE NUMBERS HANDY ☐	☐	☐	☐	☐	☐	☐

POUNDS GAINED: _____   WEIGHT: _____

QUESTIONS FOR YOUR HEALTH CARE PROVIDER:

MONTH: _____

SECOND MONTH OF PREGNANCY

SUNDAY	MONDAY	TUESDAY	WEDNESDAY	THURSDAY	FRIDAY	SATURDAY
YOU MAY EXPERIENCE MORNING SICKNESS ☐	☐	☐	☐	☐	☐	☐
☐	☐	☐	☐	☐	☐	☐
TAKE IT EASY; REST WHEN YOU CAN ☐	☐	☐	☐	☐	☐	☐
☐	☐	☐	☐	☐	☐	☐
BEGIN LIGHT ROUTINE EXERCISE (WALKING) ☐	☐	☐	☐	☐	☐	☐

POUNDS GAINED: _____   WEIGHT: _____

QUESTIONS FOR YOUR HEALTH CARE PROVIDER:

MONTH: _____

THIRD MONTH OF PREGNANCY

SUNDAY	MONDAY	TUESDAY	WEDNESDAY	THURSDAY	FRIDAY	SATURDAY
SELECT A HEALTH CARE PROVIDER; MAKE FIRST APPOINTMENT ☐	☐	☐	☐	☐	☐	☐
☐	☐	☐	BEGIN READING PREGNANCY AND CHILDBIRTH BOOKS ☐	☐	☐	☐
PLAN SPECIAL TIME WITH YOUR PARTNER ☐	☐	☐	☐	☐	☐	☐
☐	☐	☐	☐	☐	☐	☐
CONTINUE MAKING HEALTHY FOOD CHOICES ☐	☐	☐	☐	☐	☐	☐

POUNDS GAINED: _____   WEIGHT: _____

QUESTIONS FOR YOUR HEALTH CARE PROVIDER:

MONTH: _____

FOURTH MONTH OF PREGNANCY

SUNDAY	MONDAY	TUESDAY	WEDNESDAY	THURSDAY	FRIDAY	SATURDAY
☐ LET YOUR BOSS KNOW YOUR HAPPY NEWS	☐	☐	☐ TAKE A QUIET WALK EVERY DAY	☐	☐	☐
☐	☐	☐	☐	☐	☐	☐
☐ CHECK OUT YOUR INSURANCE BENEFITS	☐	☐	☐	☐	☐	☐
☐	☐	☐	☐	☐	☐	☐
☐ PLAN A BUDGET FOR BABY'S NEEDS	☐	☐ START COMPARISON SHOPPING FOR FURNITURE, ETC.	☐			☐

POUNDS GAINED: _____ WEIGHT: _____

QUESTIONS FOR YOUR HEALTH CARE PROVIDER:

MONTH: _____

FIFTH MONTH OF PREGNANCY

SUNDAY	MONDAY	TUESDAY	WEDNESDAY	THURSDAY	FRIDAY	SATURDAY
☐ PLAN A WEEKEND GETAWAY WITH YOUR PARTNER	☐	☐ START MATERNITY CLOTHES SHOPPING	☐	☐	☐	☐
☐	☐	☐	☐	☐	☐	☐
☐ DETERMINE WHAT ITEMS YOU CAN BORROW	☐	☐	☐	☐	☐	☐
☐	☐	☐	☐	☐	☐	☐
☐ FINISH COMPARISON SHOPPING—MAKE SELECTIONS	☐	☐	☐	☐	☐	☐

POUNDS GAINED:_____ WEIGHT:_____

QUESTIONS FOR YOUR HEALTH CARE PROVIDER:

MONTH: _____

SIXTH MONTH OF PREGNANCY

SUNDAY	MONDAY	TUESDAY	WEDNESDAY	THURSDAY	FRIDAY	SATURDAY
SCHEDULE CHILDBIRTH CLASSES ☐	☐	☐	☐	☐	☐	☐
☐	☐	☐	☐	☐	☐	☐
BEGIN PURCHASING NURSERY ITEMS ☐	☐	☐	☐	☐	☐	☐
☐	☐	☐	☐	☐	☐	☐
MAKE A LIST OF LAYETTE ITEMS YOU'D LIKE AS GIFTS ☐	☐	☐	SCHEDULE INFANT CARE AND BREAST-FEEDING CLASSES ☐	☐	☐	☐

POUNDS GAINED: _____ WEIGHT: _____

QUESTIONS FOR YOUR HEALTH CARE PROVIDER:

MONTH: _____

SEVENTH MONTH OF PREGNANCY

SUNDAY	MONDAY	TUESDAY	WEDNESDAY	THURSDAY	FRIDAY	SATURDAY
☐ CALL VARIOUS CHILD CARE FACILITIES AND SCHEDULE SITE VISITS	☐	☐	☐	☐	☐	☐
☐	☐	☐	☐	☐	☐	☐
☐ CONTINUE READING ABOUT CHILDBIRTH AND PARENTHOOD	☐ SHARE INFORMATION WITH YOUR PARTNER	☐	☐	☐	☐	☐
☐	☐	☐	☐	☐	☐	☐
☐ FIRM UP MATERNITY LEAVE PLANS	☐	☐	☐	☐	☐	☐

POUNDS GAINED: _____ WEIGHT: _____

QUESTIONS FOR YOUR HEALTH CARE PROVIDER:

MONTH:

EIGHTH MONTH OF PREGNANCY

SUNDAY	MONDAY	TUESDAY	WEDNESDAY	THURSDAY	FRIDAY	SATURDAY
INTERVIEW PEDIATRICIANS AND MAKE A SELECTION ☐	☐	☐	☐	☐	☐	☐
☐	☐	BEGIN CHILDBIRTH CLASSES ☐	☐	☐	☐	☐
DISCUSS BREAST/BOTTLE FEEDING WITH YOUR HEALTH CARE PROVIDER ☐	☐	☐	☐	☐	☐	☐
☐	☐	SELECT BIRTH ANNOUNCEMENT AND ADDRESS ENVELOPES ☐	☐	☐	☐	☐
REGISTER OTHER CHILDREN FOR SIBLING PREP CLASSES ☐	☐	☐	☐	☐	☐	☐

POUNDS GAINED:_____ WEIGHT:_____

QUESTIONS FOR YOUR HEALTH CARE PROVIDER:

MONTH: _____

NINTH MONTH OF PREGNANCY

SUNDAY	MONDAY	TUESDAY	WEDNESDAY	THURSDAY	FRIDAY	SATURDAY
☐ TOUR HOSPITAL AND PREREGISTER	☐	☐ PACK YOUR HOSPITAL BAGS	☐	☐	☐	☐
☐	☐	☐	☐	☐	☐	☐
☐ MAKE A LIST OF PEOPLE TO NOTIFY	☐	☐	☐ HAVE YOU SELECTED A NAME FOR YOUR BABY?	☐	☐	☐
☐	☐	☐	☐	☐	☐	☐
☐ TIE UP LOOSE ENDS AT HOME	☐	☐ FIRM UP CHILD CARE ARRANGEMENTS	☐	☐	☐ TAKE A PICTURE OF YOURSELF GOING OUT THE DOOR . . .	☐

POUNDS GAINED: _____   WEIGHT: _____

QUESTIONS FOR YOUR HEALTH CARE PROVIDER:

NOTES

NOTES

About the Author

Susan Kagen Podell is a Registered Dietitian and Certified Diabetes Educator living in Columbus, Ohio, with her husband and two young daughters. She is the author of *Vest Pocket Cholesterol Counter, Vest Pocket Fat Counter, A Guide to Eating Right During Pregnancy, The Pocket Vitamin Guide,* and *The Pocket Carbohydrate Counter.*